VITALITY GUIDE'S FIRST AID MANUAL

CPR, Wound Care, and Practical Solutions for Everyday Emergencies

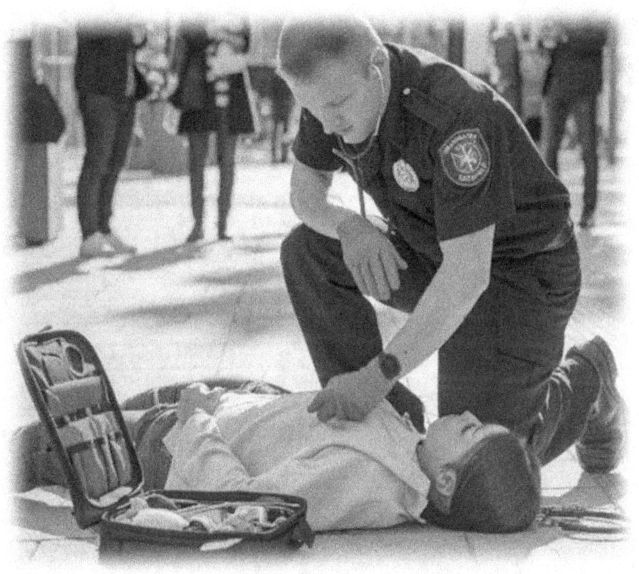

Caren Woods

Table of Contents

Introduction

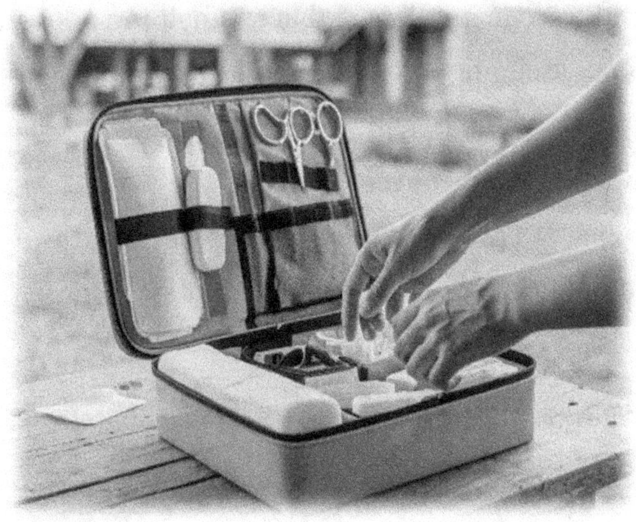

There's a certain confidence that comes from knowing you're prepared—truly prepared—not just in theory, but in a way that empowers you to face emergencies with calm and assurance. When those unexpected moments arise, the ones that can make your heart race and your mind freeze, there's a quiet strength in knowing exactly what to do. This guide, *Vitality Guide's First Aid Manual*, was created to give you that strength.

Imagine, just for a moment, what it would feel like to handle emergencies with steady hands and a clear mind. Whether it's helping a loved one, assisting a stranger, or taking care of yourself, you'll know you're equipped to act swiftly and effectively. This book is more than a collection of first aid techniques; it's a pathway to becoming someone who can offer calm in a crisis.

We often think of first aid as a set of skills we hope we never have to use. But life has a way of surprising us, and emergencies rarely come with a warning. They happen in the most ordinary settings—a family dinner, a walk around the neighborhood, or a quiet evening at home. They happen to friends, family, and even strangers who might need you in that crucial moment. And that's where your preparation comes into play.

What you'll find in these pages is a practical approach to first aid that's tailored for everyday life. You don't need a medical background or special equipment to make a difference; you just need knowledge, confidence, and the willingness to step forward. This guide will lead you through the essentials of first aid, from handling minor cuts and bruises to managing more serious injuries and illnesses.

Each chapter covers different aspects of emergency care, including:

- ***Step-by-Step Instructions:*** In a high-pressure moment, you want clarity. Each section is designed with simple, straightforward steps, guiding you from assessment to action. Whether it's applying pressure to a wound or performing CPR, you'll know exactly what to do.

- ***Specialized Guidance for All Ages:*** Emergencies don't discriminate by age, and neither does this guide. You'll find information on how to help everyone, from young children to seniors, ensuring you're prepared no matter who needs assistance.

- ***Practical Tips for Staying Calm:*** Staying calm is one of the most powerful tools you can have in an emergency. This book includes tips to help you keep your composure, assess the situation, and take the appropriate steps without letting panic take over.

- ***Tools for Building Your Own First Aid Kit:*** Having a well-stocked first aid kit is a simple but invaluable step toward readiness. This guide shows you exactly what to include, whether for your home, your car, or an outdoor adventure.

Each chapter is crafted to give you the essentials without overwhelming detail, focusing on the actions that matter most in the moments that count. From the basic to the advanced, every technique is carefully chosen to empower you with both knowledge and confidence. This isn't about memorizing endless medical terminology or reading through complicated procedures. It's about putting essential, lifesaving knowledge directly into your hands.

Let's face it: the unexpected can be intimidating. But that's precisely why preparation is so important. Imagine being able to keep calm as you assess a broken bone or help someone through an allergic reaction. Picture yourself responding with confidence to a situation you once thought beyond your abilities. That's the kind of empowerment this book aims to provide.

Think of this guide as a toolkit—a trusted resource you can turn to again and again. The more you engage with these pages, the more natural it will feel to respond quickly and effectively when the need arises. And as you progress, you'll begin to feel a shift. You'll find yourself thinking differently, acting with greater calm, and realizing just how capable you really are.

In these pages, you'll encounter scenarios you may have never thought about before—injuries, medical emergencies, and other urgent situations. But by reading through them, practicing the techniques, and reflecting on your own readiness, you're building a powerful foundation. You're choosing to be someone who is ready, someone who can bring reassurance and aid when it's needed most.

The skills in this guide are timeless, useful not only in emergency situations but in everyday life. They're not only about providing care in urgent moments; they're about cultivating a sense of security and capability. Even if you never have to use these techniques, the peace of mind they bring is invaluable. And if you do, you'll know you have the knowledge to make a real difference.

So here's to you, the reader, and your journey into becoming more prepared, more resilient, and more empowered. As you turn each page, remember that you're not just learning first aid; you're embracing a proactive approach to life and safety. This book is your ally, guiding you step-by-step toward readiness, and it's an honor to be part of that journey with you.

Welcome to *Vitality Guide's First Aid Manual*.

Chapter 1: Introduction to First Aid

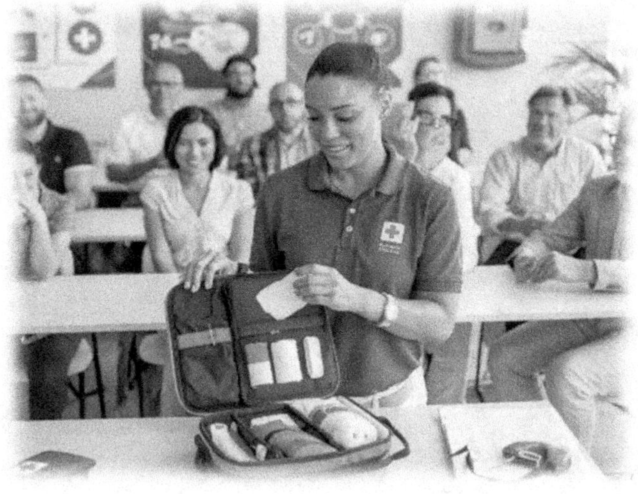

Sylvia, a hiking guide, sprang into action when one of her clients slipped and severely cut her leg. Sylvia calmly assessed the wound, stopped the bleeding, and applied a pressure bandage. She then called for emergency assistance and kept her client calm until help arrived. Thanks to Sylvia's first aid training, the client received timely medical attention and made a full recovery. Sylvia's quick thinking and confidence demonstrated the importance of basic first aid knowledge in emergency situations, saving lives and reducing the risk of long-term damage.

The Importance of First Aid in Everyday Life

First aid plays a vital role in everyday life, providing essential skills that can save lives and prevent further injury. Understanding the basics of first aid equips you with the knowledge and confidence to respond effectively in emergencies, whether at home, work, or in public settings. This foundational skill not only helps individuals but also fosters a safer community.

When accidents happen, having first aid skills allows you to act quickly and appropriately. Immediate response can significantly influence the outcome of an injury or medical condition. For example, knowing how to administer CPR in case someone collapses can be the difference between life and death. Furthermore, first aid knowledge empowers you to handle various situations, such as minor cuts, burns, or allergic reactions, preventing complications and ensuring that help is sought when needed.

In many cases, emergencies are unpredictable. They can occur at any time and in any place, making it crucial for everyone to be prepared. Understanding first aid is not just for medical professionals; it is a skill that everyone can learn. Whether you're a parent, teacher, or simply a member of the community, knowing how to provide basic first aid can enhance safety for those around you. For instance, if your child gets a scrape while playing outside, having first aid knowledge enables you to treat it quickly and effectively, reducing the risk of infection.

First aid also plays a key role in fostering a sense of community responsibility. When more people are trained in first aid, the likelihood of effective assistance increases during emergencies. This collective preparedness can create a safer environment where individuals feel more secure, knowing that help is readily available in times of crisis. Communities with a higher number of first aid-trained individuals tend to respond better to emergencies, leading to quicker recovery and better overall outcomes.

In addition to practical skills, understanding the principles of first aid can reduce panic in emergency situations. Many people feel anxious when faced with an unexpected medical event. However, with basic first aid training, you can approach the situation with confidence and a clear mind. This calmness can help those around you feel more secure and focused. For example, if a colleague experiences a sudden health issue, knowing how to assess the situation and provide immediate help can minimize chaos and enable faster access to professional medical assistance.

Moreover, first aid training also encompasses legal and ethical considerations. Knowing your rights and responsibilities when providing first aid can guide your actions and help you feel more comfortable stepping in during emergencies. For instance, "Good Samaritan" laws protect individuals who assist others in emergency situations, ensuring that you won't face legal repercussions as long as you act within your training and capabilities. This understanding encourages more people to take action when they see someone in need.

First aid training is accessible to everyone. Many organizations offer courses that cater to various skill levels, from basic first aid to advanced life support. These courses often include hands-on practice, allowing you to learn in a supportive environment. By participating in first aid training, you not only gain valuable skills but also contribute to a culture of safety and preparedness. Additionally, some workplaces may require first aid certification for employees, further emphasizing its importance in professional settings.

Extra Tips:

-Consider taking a first aid course to build your confidence and skills.

-Keep a well-stocked first aid kit at home and in your car.

-Review first aid techniques regularly to keep your knowledge fresh.

-Teach family members about basic first aid to create a supportive network in emergencies.

Basic Principles of First Aid and Emergency Response

First aid is essential in emergencies, providing immediate care to those who are injured or ill before professional help arrives. Understanding basic principles of first aid not only empowers you to help others but also can save lives. This section will cover key principles and practical steps you can take in emergency situations.

The foundation of first aid rests on several basic principles that guide your actions during emergencies. First, always prioritize your safety and the safety of others. Before assisting anyone, make sure the environment is safe. For instance, if there's a fire, explosion, or ongoing traffic hazard, don't rush in without assessing the situation. You cannot help someone if you become a victim yourself. Once you have ensured safety, you can begin to evaluate the situation and provide assistance.

The next principle is to assess the casualty. This means observing the person's condition and determining what kind of help they need. Start with a primary survey, which includes checking for responsiveness, breathing, and circulation. Approach the person calmly, and if they are unconscious or unable to respond, gently shake their shoulders and ask if they can hear you. If they don't respond, check for breathing by looking for chest movements or listening for breath sounds.

If the person is breathing but unresponsive, place them in the recovery position. This involves rolling them onto their side while ensuring their airway remains clear, which helps prevent choking. If the person is not breathing, you will need to perform CPR immediately, so be prepared to initiate this life-saving procedure if necessary.

After performing a primary survey, you should conduct a secondary survey to gather more detailed information about the person's condition. Ask the casualty about their injuries or symptoms if they are conscious. This can provide valuable information for emergency responders. Look for visible injuries, such as cuts, bruises, or fractures, and check for any medical alert tags that might indicate pre-existing conditions like diabetes or allergies.

Once you have assessed the situation, it is crucial to prioritize care. This means determining which injuries need immediate attention. Triage is a method used in emergencies to sort patients based on the severity of their condition. If you encounter multiple casualties, focus on those whose lives are at risk first. For instance, someone who is bleeding heavily or not breathing should receive care before someone with a minor injury.

The next essential principle is to provide the appropriate first aid for the injuries you've identified. This could involve controlling bleeding, treating burns, or immobilizing fractures. For bleeding, apply direct pressure to the wound with a clean cloth or bandage. If the bleeding doesn't stop, maintain pressure and consider elevating the injured area above the heart to help reduce blood flow. For burns, cool the area with running water for at least ten minutes and cover it with a sterile dressing.

Communication is another critical principle of first aid. If you have others around you, delegate tasks where possible. For example, ask someone to call emergency services while you attend to the injured person. Make sure to provide them with all necessary information, such as the nature of the injury and the person's condition. If you're alone, it's essential to call for help yourself before starting any treatment. This way, professional help can arrive while you provide care.

Documentation is often overlooked but is essential in first aid situations. If possible, keep a record of what you have observed, the care you provided, and the time each action was taken. This information can be vital for medical professionals when they arrive, ensuring they understand the situation fully.

Once you've provided care and called for help, stay with the injured person until emergency services arrive. Monitor their condition continuously. Be prepared to offer reassurance, as injuries can be frightening. Providing emotional support can help keep the casualty calm and can also assist in maintaining their stability until further help arrives.

Understanding the legal and ethical considerations surrounding first aid is also essential. You should always act within your abilities and knowledge. If you provide care, do so to the best of your abilities. In many regions, Good Samaritan laws protect those who assist in emergencies from legal repercussions, provided that the care was given in good faith and without gross negligence.

To summarize, knowing the basic principles of first aid empowers you to respond effectively in emergencies. Always prioritize your safety, assess the situation, provide appropriate care, communicate clearly, and document your actions. Being prepared can make a significant difference in the outcome for someone in need.

Extra Tips:

-Consider taking a certified first aid course to gain hands-on experience.

-Keep a well-stocked first aid kit accessible in your home and car.

-Regularly review first aid techniques to stay fresh on your skills and knowledge.

Legal and Ethical Considerations in First Aid

When you step in to provide first aid, understanding the legal and ethical considerations is crucial. Not only do these aspects protect you, but they also ensure that the person in need receives appropriate care. First aid is a critical intervention, and it's essential to be aware of your rights and responsibilities as a responder. This section explores the legal implications of giving first aid, the ethical principles guiding your actions, and how to navigate potential challenges you may face.

Legal Considerations

One of the primary legal concepts in first aid is the Good Samaritan law, which protects individuals who provide assistance in emergency situations. These laws vary by location but generally protect you from liability if you act in good faith to help someone in need. Here are a few key points to remember about Good Samaritan laws:

1. **Acting Reasonably**: You are protected when you provide aid as long as your actions are reasonable and based on your level of training. For example, if you have basic first aid training, performing CPR on someone who has collapsed is within your scope of practice. However, performing advanced procedures that you're not trained to do may expose you to liability.

2. **Consent**: Before administering first aid, it's important to obtain consent from the injured person if they are conscious and capable of giving it. If the person is unconscious and unable to respond, it is generally assumed that they would want help. In some cases, such as with minors, you may need consent from a parent or guardian.

3. **Duty to Act:** If you are trained in first aid and you encounter a situation where someone is injured or in distress, you may have a legal duty to act. This duty varies by location and can be influenced by your profession. For example,

healthcare professionals have a legal obligation to provide care.

4. Documentation: Keeping a record of your actions can protect you legally. Document the details of the incident, including what you observed, the care you provided, and the time you arrived on the scene. This information can be crucial if any questions arise later about the care you provided.

Ethical Considerations

Alongside legal aspects, ethical considerations play a significant role in how you provide first aid. Here are some fundamental ethical principles to keep in mind:

1. Beneficence: This principle emphasizes the importance of doing good and acting in the best interest of the patient. When providing first aid, your primary goal is to help the person in need. You should focus on delivering care that maximizes their well-being and minimizes harm.

2. Non-Maleficence: Often summarized as "do no harm," this principle highlights the importance of avoiding actions that could worsen the person's condition. Before taking any steps, assess the situation carefully and ensure your actions do not cause further injury.

3. Autonomy: Respecting a person's autonomy means acknowledging their right to make decisions about their own care. This includes their right to refuse treatment. If someone declines your help, you must respect their decision, provided they are competent to make such choices.

4. Justice: This principle involves treating all individuals fairly and providing care without discrimination. Regardless of the person's background, ensure that everyone receives the same level of assistance. It's important to focus on the individual's needs, not their circumstances.

Navigating Challenges

Providing first aid can present challenges, especially in complex situations. Here are some strategies to navigate these difficulties effectively:

1. Stay Calm: Your demeanor can significantly impact the situation. Remaining calm helps you think clearly and provides reassurance to the person needing help. Take a deep breath and focus on the task at hand.

2. Communicate Clearly: When interacting with the injured person or bystanders, use clear and simple language. Explain what you are doing and why, which can help alleviate anxiety and build trust.

3. Work as a Team: If other people are present, delegate tasks to them to manage the situation more effectively. For instance, ask someone to call emergency services while you attend to the person in need.

4. Know Your Limits: Recognize your training and expertise. If the situation escalates beyond your skills, it's important to seek professional medical help as soon as possible.

5. Continuous Learning: Stay updated on first aid practices and legal guidelines. Regularly refresh your knowledge and skills through courses and training sessions. This will ensure you are prepared to respond effectively and confidently in emergencies.

Extra Tips:

Always carry a first aid manual or guide with you. Familiarize yourself with local laws regarding first aid to ensure you are informed about your rights and responsibilities. Additionally, consider taking refresher courses to stay updated on the latest first aid techniques and protocols.

Chapter 2: Assessing the Situation

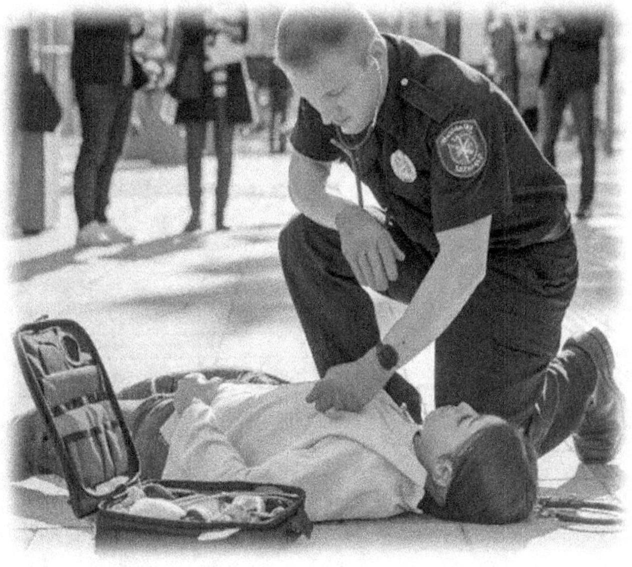

When a sudden storm capsized Ben's kayak, he remained calm and assessed his situation. He evaluated his injuries, checked for hazards, and took stock of his equipment. Recognizing the danger of hypothermia, Ben prioritized finding shelter and starting a fire. Using his emergency whistle to signal for help, he then used his navigation skills to guide rescuers to his location. Thanks to Ben's thorough assessment and clear thinking, he was rescued within hours, shaken but unharmed. Ben's effective assessment demonstrated the critical importance of staying calm and evaluating situations accurately in emergency situations.

Performing a Primary Survey: DRSABCD

When you encounter a medical emergency, the first step is to assess the situation and ensure the safety of yourself and others. This is where the DRSABCD approach comes into play. Understanding and executing this primary survey method can save lives by guiding you through critical steps needed to address potential dangers and assess the victim's condition. This guide will break down each component of DRSABCD, ensuring you feel confident and prepared to take action when it matters most.

The DRSABCD acronym stands for Danger, Response, Send for help, Airway, Breathing, Circulation, and Disability. Each letter represents a vital step in assessing the situation and providing first aid effectively.

Danger is the first thing to check. Before approaching the victim, you need to ensure the area is safe for both you prnd the person in need.

Look around for any potential hazards such as traffic, fire, electrical wires, or aggressive individuals. If the scene is not safe, do not put yourself at risk. You might need to move the person to a safer location if possible. Your safety is paramount, as you cannot help anyone if you become a victim yourself.

Next, assess the Response of the person in distress. Gently shake their shoulders and loudly ask if they are okay. This helps determine their level of consciousness. If they respond, that's a good sign; however, you should still monitor their condition closely. If there is no response, it indicates a more serious situation, and you should move to the next steps quickly.

Once you establish that the person is unresponsive, the next action is to send for help. Call emergency services immediately or ask someone else nearby to do so. Provide clear information about the location and the situation. This step is crucial because professional medical help will be on the way, allowing you to focus on caring for the individual. While waiting for help to arrive, it's essential to proceed with the next steps in the survey.

The next components of DRSABCD focus on the physical state of the victim, starting with checking the Airway. An open airway is critical for the victim's survival. If the person is unresponsive, you need to tilt their head back gently to open the airway. You can do this by placing one hand on their forehead and using your other hand to lift their chin. This position helps prevent the tongue from blocking the throat, allowing for air passage.

After ensuring the airway is clear, it's time to check for breathing. Look, listen, and feel for any signs of breathing for about 10 seconds. Look for the rise and fall of the chest, listen for breath sounds, and feel for air from their nose or mouth. If the person is breathing normally, you should monitor their condition closely until help arrives. If they are not breathing or breathing abnormally, you need to start CPR immediately.

Next in the sequence is Circulation. This step involves checking for signs of circulation, such as a pulse. For adults, you can check the carotid artery located on the side of the neck. For infants, check the brachial artery on the inside of the arm. If you cannot detect a pulse, begin chest compressions as part of CPR. Aim for a depth of about 2 inches for adults, and for infants, use two fingers to push down about 1.5 inches at a rate of 100 to 120 compressions per minute.

Finally, the last step is assessing Disability. This involves checking the level of consciousness and responsiveness. You can use the AVPU scale: Alert, Voice, Pain, and Unresponsive. This assessment gives a quick snapshot of the individual's neurological status. If they are unresponsive, this indicates a serious condition, and it's crucial to keep monitoring their breathing and circulation until professional help arrives.

Once you've completed the primary survey, it's essential to remain with the individual, providing reassurance and monitoring their condition. You should also be prepared to update emergency responders on what you observed during the survey, as this information can be crucial for their treatment.

Extra Tips:

Always remember to stay calm and focused during an emergency. Practice the DRSABCD method regularly so it becomes second nature. Consider taking a first aid course to improve your skills and knowledge, which will prepare you to respond confidently in any situation. Familiarize yourself with common emergencies and appropriate first aid responses, as this will enhance your ability to act swiftly when needed.

Conducting a Secondary Survey for Injuries

When someone is injured, your first action should always be to assess whether they are in immediate danger. Once any life-threatening issues are managed, such as breathing difficulties or severe bleeding, you can conduct a secondary survey. This step is crucial for identifying and addressing other injuries the person may have sustained. The secondary survey helps gather more information, allowing you to provide better assistance or communicate effectively with emergency responders.

To start the secondary survey, ensure the scene is safe, and the person is stable. Introduce yourself and explain what you are going to do to keep them calm. Always obtain consent before touching someone, unless they are unconscious or unable to give consent. If possible, ask about their medical history, allergies, or medications, as this information can be vital for treatment.

Begin your survey with a head-to-toe examination. You want to check for any visible injuries, such as cuts, bruises, or swelling. Look for signs of pain or discomfort as you gently palpate or press on different areas of the body. Always start at the head and work your way down to ensure a systematic approach.

Head and Neck: Begin by examining the head and neck area. Check for any swelling, cuts, or bruises. Look for any signs of bleeding from the scalp or face. Gently press on the skull to identify any fractures or deformities. Assess the neck for any stiffness or pain that may indicate a spinal injury. If the person has any visible wounds or swelling, be cautious when moving their head or neck.

Chest and Abdomen: Next, assess the chest. Look for any signs of bruising, open wounds, or difficulty breathing. If the person is having trouble breathing, encourage them to sit up or find a position that feels more comfortable. Gently press on the chest to check for any abnormalities, like broken ribs. After checking the chest, move to the abdomen. Observe for any distension or swelling. Gently palpate the abdomen, starting from the lower quadrants and working your way up. Be aware of any signs of pain or tenderness, as these may indicate internal injuries.

Arms and Hands: Continue the survey by examining the arms and hands. Look for cuts, bruises, or deformities. Check the range of motion by having the person move their arms if they can. Ask about any pain they feel during movement, as this can help pinpoint injuries like fractures or sprains.

Legs and Feet: Next, inspect the legs and feet. Similar to the arms, observe for any visible injuries. Ask the person to wiggle their toes and move their legs. Look for signs of swelling or deformity, which can indicate fractures or dislocations. Be mindful of the person's comfort level and avoid causing them further pain.

Vital Signs: As you conduct the secondary survey, pay attention to the person's vital signs, including their pulse, breathing rate, and level of consciousness. A change in these indicators can signify worsening conditions. For example, if the person's breathing becomes shallow or rapid, it may indicate a need for immediate medical attention. If they lose consciousness, be prepared to perform CPR if necessary.

Once the survey is complete, document your findings. Make notes of any visible injuries, complaints of pain, and changes in vital signs. This information is critical for emergency responders when they arrive on the scene. If the person is conscious and able to communicate, ask them questions about how the injury occurred, their symptoms, and any medical history that could be relevant.

If you identify any serious injuries during your secondary survey, prioritize addressing them based on the severity. For instance, if a person has a fractured limb and is also showing signs of shock, you must manage the shock first before addressing the fracture.

Finally, keep the injured person as calm and comfortable as possible while you wait for professional help to arrive. Reassure them that help is on the way and avoid giving them anything to eat or drink, as this may complicate medical treatment.

Conducting a thorough secondary survey is an essential skill in first aid. It allows you to gather vital information and provide the necessary care for any injuries sustained. Remember that each injury is unique, and your survey should be adaptable based on the situation.

Extra Tips:

Always keep your first aid kit handy during emergencies to address various injuries as needed. Practice your skills regularly so that they become second nature. Familiarizing yourself with the signs and symptoms of common injuries can also help you conduct a more effective survey. Staying calm and reassuring can greatly impact the injured person's emotional state, making your role in providing first aid even more effective.

Prioritizing Care: Triage in First Aid

When you're faced with a situation where multiple individuals need first aid, knowing how to prioritize care is crucial. Triage is the process of determining the urgency of medical needs so that those who need help the most receive it first. This approach can make a significant difference in outcomes during emergencies, especially when resources are limited. Understanding how to effectively assess and prioritize injuries can help you provide the best possible care.

Understanding Triage

Triage originates from the French word "trier," which means "to sort." In the context of first aid, it refers to categorizing patients based on the severity of their injuries. This method ensures that those in critical condition are treated before those with less severe issues. Triage is vital in emergencies like natural disasters, mass casualty incidents, or situations where multiple people are injured simultaneously.

When you arrive at the scene, take a moment to assess the situation. Look for any potential dangers, such as ongoing hazards or unstable environments. Your safety is paramount; only then can you assist others effectively.

The Triage Process

1. Initial Assessment: Start by quickly evaluating the scene. Check for immediate dangers and ensure it is safe for you to provide aid. Once you're safe, look at each individual who needs help.

2. Categorization: Use the following categories to classify injuries based on urgency:

Immediate (Red): These individuals need urgent medical attention. They may have life-threatening conditions such as severe bleeding, difficulty breathing, or unconsciousness. Treat these patients first.

Delayed (Yellow): These patients have serious injuries that are not immediately life-threatening. They require medical attention but can wait a bit longer. Examples include broken bones or significant wounds that are not actively bleeding.

Minor (Green): These individuals have non-life-threatening injuries. They might have cuts or bruises that don't require immediate care. If possible, give them instructions on how to care for themselves while you tend to those who need urgent help.

Deceased (Black): Unfortunately, some individuals may be beyond help. If someone has no pulse, is not breathing, and shows no signs of life, it is vital to assess the situation quickly and move on to assist others who can still be saved.

3. **Communication**: As you assess and categorize, communicate your findings with other responders or bystanders. This is crucial if you have a team assisting you. Let them know who needs immediate care and assign tasks

accordingly. If you are alone, try to call for help or ask someone else to alert emergency services.

4. Provide Care: Once you've prioritized the injured, begin treating those in the Immediate category. Focus on stopping any life-threatening bleeding, ensuring the airway is clear, and providing CPR if necessary. After addressing those in immediate need, move on to the Delayed category, and finally to the Minor injuries.

5. Reassess: Situations can change quickly. Continuously reassess the condition of the individuals you're helping. If someone's condition worsens, they may need to be moved to a higher priority category.

Special Considerations

In triage, it's also essential to be aware of special populations, like children, elderly individuals, or those with disabilities. These individuals may require extra attention, as their conditions might not be immediately apparent. Always assess the situation holistically and consider the potential for hidden injuries.

Furthermore, if you're in a large-scale emergency with multiple victims, you may encounter the need to use your judgment about the resources available. In some cases, you might have to make tough decisions about who receives care first based on their condition and the likelihood of survival.

After the Emergency

Once the immediate crisis has passed, it's essential to ensure that all individuals receive proper follow-up care. After providing initial first aid, document your actions and the conditions of the injured. This information can be invaluable for emergency responders when they arrive.

Extra Tips

-Always carry a first aid kit that includes tools for triage, such as bandages and gauze, to manage injuries effectively.

-Consider taking a certified first aid and CPR course to enhance your skills and confidence in handling emergencies.

-Practice triaging in scenarios to become more comfortable with the process, allowing you to react swiftly and effectively in real-life situations.

Understanding triage and prioritizing care can make a significant difference when lives are at stake. With practice and knowledge, you can be prepared to make critical decisions that could save lives in emergencies.

Chapter 3: Cardiopulmonary Resuscitation (CPR)

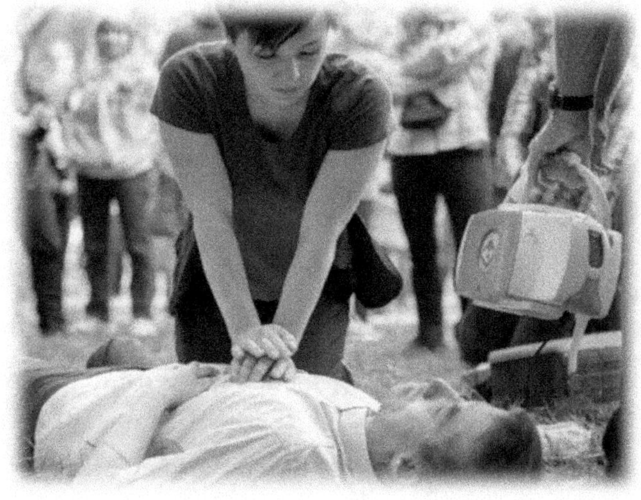

While jogging, Mark witnessed a fellow runner collapse from cardiac arrest. Without hesitation, Mark began CPR, administering chest compressions and rescue breaths. He continued until paramedics arrived, thanks to a bystander's 911 call. Mark's timely and proper CPR technique helped maintain blood flow to the victim's brain and heart, significantly increasing chances of survival. The runner was revived at the hospital and made a full recovery. Mark's lifesaving actions demonstrated the critical importance of knowing CPR, emphasizing that anyone can make a difference in a cardiac emergency.

CPR for Adults: Technique and Timing

Knowing how to perform CPR (cardiopulmonary resuscitation) can be a lifesaver. In emergencies where someone's heart has stopped or they are not breathing, your quick actions can make a significant difference. This section will guide you through the techniques and timing of CPR for adults, equipping you with the essential skills to respond effectively.

To start, it's crucial to understand when CPR is needed. You should perform CPR if an adult is unresponsive and not breathing or only gasping. Always call emergency services immediately before starting CPR. If you're alone, call for help first; if someone else is present, have them call while you attend to the victim.

Performing CPR: The Technique

1. Check the Scene and the Victim: Before approaching, ensure the area is safe for you and the victim. Check the person for responsiveness by gently shaking their shoulders and asking loudly if they are okay. If there's no response, proceed with CPR.

2. Position the Victim: Carefully roll the person onto their back. Make sure they are on a firm, flat surface. If the victim is in water, pull them out if it's safe to do so.

3. Open the Airway: Tilt the victim's head back slightly by placing one hand on their forehead and using two fingers from your other hand to lift the chin. This position opens the airway, allowing for better airflow.

4. Check for Breathing: Look, listen, and feel for breathing for no more than 10 seconds. If the person is not breathing or only gasping, you need to start CPR.

5. Start Chest Compressions: Kneel beside the person and place the heel of one hand on the center of their chest, just below the nipple line. Place your other hand on top of the first and interlock your fingers. Keep your elbows straight and use your body weight to push down hard and fast. Aim for a compression depth of about two inches, allowing the chest to fully recoil between compressions. The rate should be 100 to 120 compressions per minute. Remember, it's essential to push hard and fast, but you should also keep a rhythm that can help you maintain speed. You can use a song with a steady beat, like "Stayin' Alive" by the Bee Gees, to help keep the right tempo.

6. Give Rescue Breaths: After 30 compressions, you will give two rescue breaths. To do this, again open the airway by tilting the head back slightly. Pinch the nose shut, take a normal breath, and seal your lips around the victim's mouth. Give a breath that lasts about one second, watching for the chest to rise. Repeat this for a second breath, allowing the chest to fall back down in between.

7. Continue the Cycle: Alternate between 30 chest compressions and two rescue breaths.

Keep doing this until emergency personnel arrive or the person starts to show signs of life, such as moving, breathing normally, or coughing.

Timing is Crucial

The effectiveness of CPR is heavily influenced by how quickly you respond. The sooner you begin compressions, the better the chance of survival for the person in distress. Aim to start CPR within a few minutes of the victim collapsing. If you can access an AED (automated external defibrillator), use it as soon as possible. It can help restore a normal heart rhythm and increase the likelihood of a successful outcome.

If you're unsure about giving rescue breaths, it's perfectly acceptable to perform "hands-only CPR," which involves continuous chest compressions without rescue breaths. Studies show that hands-only CPR can be just as effective in many cases, especially when you are not trained or feel uncomfortable with the rescue breaths.

Monitoring Your Progress

Keep an eye on the victim for any changes. If they regain consciousness, turn them onto their side in the recovery position if it's safe to do so. This position helps keep the airway clear in case they vomit or have difficulty breathing.

Extra Tips

Before you leave, remember these extra tips for CPR. Always seek training through certified organizations to keep your skills fresh and up-to-date. Regularly review the CPR guidelines and practice the technique so you feel confident in an emergency. Also, consider carrying a CPR mask in your first aid kit to help protect yourself when giving rescue breaths. Practicing CPR can save lives, and being prepared is the key to making a difference when it counts.

CPR for Children and Infants: Adjusting Your Approach

Performing CPR on children and infants is crucial, as their bodies are different from adults in terms of size and physiology. Understanding these differences can make a significant impact on outcomes in emergencies. In this section, you'll learn how to adjust your CPR techniques for younger individuals, ensuring you provide the most effective care possible.

When it comes to CPR for children and infants, the first thing to remember is that their airways, hearts, and overall anatomy differ significantly from adults. Children have smaller airways, making them more susceptible to obstruction. Additionally, the chest of a child or infant is softer, requiring less force when performing chest compressions. Therefore, it's essential to adjust your technique based on the age and size of the child.

Before you start CPR, it's crucial to ensure the scene is safe. Approach the child calmly, and if you're not alone, ask someone else to call for emergency services. If you're alone with an infant, it's okay to perform CPR for about two minutes before calling for help, as infants can deteriorate quickly. For older children, if they are unresponsive, call for help right away, then begin CPR.

Performing CPR on Infants

When doing CPR on infants (typically under one year old), the technique differs from that used for older children and adults. Start by ensuring the infant is lying on a firm, flat surface. If the infant is unresponsive and not breathing, follow these steps:

1. **Check Responsiveness**: Gently tap the infant and shout to see if they respond. If they do not, proceed to the next steps.

2. **Call for Help**: If you are alone, give two minutes of care before calling emergency services.

3. Positioning: Place the infant on their back on a firm surface. Make sure the head is in a neutral position to maintain an open airway.

4. Open the Airway: Use the head-tilt, chin-lift method by placing one hand on the forehead and using your other hand to gently lift the chin. Be careful not to tilt the head too far back, as this may close off the airway.

5. Check for Breathing: Look for chest movement, listen for breath sounds, or feel for air on your cheek for no more than 10 seconds. If the infant is not breathing normally, it's time to give rescue breaths.

6. Rescue Breaths: Cover the infant's mouth and nose with your mouth, ensuring a good seal. Give two gentle breaths, each lasting about one second, watching for the chest to rise as you do so.

7. Chest Compressions: For infants, use two fingers placed just below the nipple line on the breastbone. Press down firmly and quickly, at a rate of 100 to 120 compressions per minute. Compress the chest about 1.5 inches deep, allowing it to fully recoil between compressions. Alternate between 30 chest compressions and 2 rescue breaths.

Performing CPR on Children

For children aged one to puberty, you will adjust your technique further:

1. **Check Responsiveness**: Just as with infants, gently shake the child and shout to check for responsiveness.

2. **Call for Help**: If the child does not respond and is not breathing normally, call for emergency help immediately.

3. **Positioning**: Lay the child flat on their back on a firm surface.

4. **Open the Airway**: Use the head-tilt, chin-lift method, just as you would for an infant but with a slight tilt back.

5. Check for Breathing: Look, listen, and feel for normal breathing for up to 10 seconds. If the child is not breathing, you will proceed to give rescue breaths.

6. Rescue Breaths: Pinch the nose shut, cover the child's mouth with yours, and give two breaths that last about one second each, ensuring the chest rises.

7. Chest Compressions: For children, use one hand if they are larger and two hands for smaller children, pressing down on the center of the chest. Compress the chest about 2 inches deep, at a rate of 100 to 120 compressions per minute. Again, follow the pattern of 30 chest compressions to 2 rescue breaths.

In both cases, keep a close eye on the child or infant's response. If they begin to show signs of life—such as breathing or movement—stop CPR and monitor their condition until help arrives.

Lastly, always remember that performing CPR is better than doing nothing at all. Even if you feel uncertain about your technique, your efforts could save a life.

Extra Tips:

Always keep your cool in emergencies. Regularly practice CPR techniques to build confidence, and consider enrolling in a certified CPR course to stay updated on the latest practices. Having a first aid kit and knowing how to use its contents can also be beneficial during emergencies.

Using an Automated External Defibrillator (AED)

Understanding how to use an Automated External Defibrillator (AED) can be a lifesaver in emergencies. An AED is a portable device that can analyze the heart's rhythm and, if necessary, deliver an electric shock to help restore a normal heartbeat. Knowing how to operate this device is essential, especially in situations where someone is experiencing a sudden cardiac arrest. Let's explore how you can effectively use an AED to provide critical assistance.

Using an AED is straightforward, but there are a few steps to remember. First, ensure the area is safe for both you and the victim. If the person is unresponsive and not breathing, you need to call emergency services immediately or have someone else do it while you prepare to use the AED. Many AEDs are designed to give verbal prompts, guiding you through each step, so don't worry if you're unsure of what to do.

Once the AED arrives, the first thing you should do is turn it on. Most devices have a power button that is clearly marked. As soon as you power it up, the AED will begin to give you instructions. Listen carefully and follow the prompts closely. The AED will tell you to attach the pads to the person's chest. These pads are crucial because they will detect the heart's rhythm and deliver the shock if needed.

Next, you'll need to expose the person's chest. If the victim is wearing a shirt, you must remove it to ensure the pads can stick directly to the skin. If the chest is wet or hairy, dry it off or use the AED's pads to remove excess moisture. Some AEDs come with specialized pads designed for use on hairy chests, which can be very helpful. Once the chest is ready, take the pads out of their packaging and peel off the backing. Place one pad on the upper right chest, just below the collarbone, and the other pad on the lower left side of the chest, a few inches below the armpit.

After placing the pads, the AED will analyze the heart's rhythm. Make sure no one is touching the person during this analysis, as this could interfere with the readings. The AED will instruct you to stand clear while it evaluates whether a shock is needed. If the device determines that a shock is appropriate, it will charge up and instruct you to ensure everyone is clear before delivering the shock.

When you hear the AED tell you to press the shock button, do so immediately. This shock can help restore a normal rhythm to the heart. After the shock is delivered, the AED will prompt you to continue CPR. This is essential because even if the shock helps, the person may still need additional support until medical professionals arrive. If you are trained in CPR, perform it immediately after the shock. Continue to follow the AED's prompts and perform CPR until emergency responders arrive or the person starts showing signs of life, such as breathing.

It's also important to remember that an AED is safe to use. They are designed to be user-friendly and can be used on adults, children, and infants with special pediatric pads, if available. If you're using an AED on a child or an infant, make sure to use pads specifically designed for smaller bodies to ensure effectiveness and safety.

It's worth taking the time to familiarize yourself with these devices, as knowing how to use one can empower you to save a life when it matters most.

Extra Tips:

Always check the AED for maintenance and ensure it has been regularly serviced. Make sure the pads are not expired and that the device is functioning correctly. If you're in a public area, don't hesitate to ask someone nearby for help. They may be able to assist in calling for emergency services or finding an AED. Lastly, consider taking a first aid and CPR course to gain confidence and skills in emergency situations.

Chapter 4: Dealing with Bleeding and Wounds

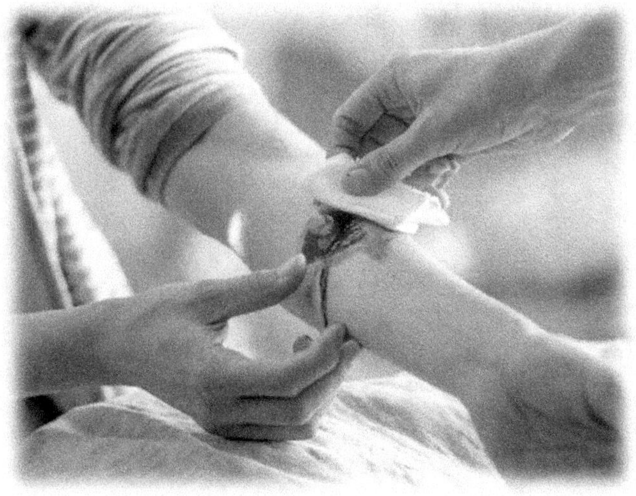

While hiking, Darlene's friend, Alex, severely cut her leg on a rocky outcropping. Darlene sprang into action, applying direct pressure to the wound and elevating Alex's leg. She then cleaned and dressed the wound with supplies from her first aid kit, stemming the bleeding. As they awaited rescue, Darlene monitored Alex's vital signs and kept her calm. Thanks to

Darlene's prompt and proper wound care, Alex received minimal scarring and made a swift recovery. Darlene's quick thinking demonstrated the importance of effective bleeding control and wound management in preventing infection and promoting healing.

Types of Bleeding: Identifying Severity

Understanding the types of bleeding and how to identify their severity is crucial for providing effective first aid. This knowledge can help you respond quickly and appropriately in emergency situations. Whether it's a minor cut or a severe injury, recognizing the type of bleeding can save lives. Here, we'll explore the various types of bleeding, how to assess their severity, and the steps to take for effective first aid.

Bleeding can be classified into three main types: arterial, venous, and capillary. Each type has distinct characteristics and requires different approaches for management.

Arterial Bleeding

Arterial bleeding is often the most severe type. It occurs when an artery is damaged, causing bright red blood to spurt out in rhythm with the heartbeat. This type of bleeding can be life-threatening because arteries carry oxygen-rich blood from the heart to the rest of the body. If you notice that someone is bleeding profusely from a wound and the blood is bright red and pulsing, this may indicate arterial bleeding.

To manage arterial bleeding, your first action should be to call for emergency assistance immediately. While waiting for help, you can take the following steps:

1. **Apply Direct Pressure**: Use a clean cloth or your hands to apply firm, direct pressure to the wound. This helps slow down the bleeding.

2. **Elevate the Injury**: If possible, raise the injured area above the level of the heart. This can help reduce blood flow to the wound.

3. **Use a Tourniquet if Necessary:** If direct pressure does not stop the bleeding and the injury is severe, you may need to use a tourniquet. This should be placed above the wound and tightened until the bleeding stops. Make sure to note the time the tourniquet was

applied, as it should be released only by medical professionals.

Venous Bleeding

Venous bleeding occurs when a vein is injured. The blood that flows from a vein is usually darker and flows steadily, rather than spurting. While venous bleeding is typically less severe than arterial bleeding, it can still be significant, especially if it involves a large vein. If someone has a cut or wound with dark red blood oozing steadily, you may be dealing with venous bleeding.

To manage venous bleeding, follow these steps:

1. Apply Direct Pressure: Like with arterial bleeding, your first action should be to apply firm, direct pressure to the wound using a clean cloth or bandage.

2. Elevate the Injury: Raising the injured area can help slow down the bleeding.

3. Monitor for Signs of Shock: Keep an eye on the injured person for signs of shock, such as pale skin, rapid breathing, or confusion. If any of these symptoms develop, it's crucial to call for emergency help immediately.

Capillary Bleeding

Capillary bleeding is the most common and least severe type of bleeding. It happens when small blood vessels are damaged, leading to slow, oozing blood. This type of bleeding is often seen with minor cuts, scrapes, or abrasions. The blood is usually a bright red color and will flow gently from the wound.

Managing capillary bleeding is straightforward:

1. Clean the Wound: Gently rinse the wound with clean water to remove any dirt or debris.

2. Apply a Bandage: After cleaning, cover the wound with a sterile bandage or adhesive strip. This helps protect it from infection and promotes healing.

3. Monitor the Injury: Keep an eye on the wound for signs of infection, such as increased redness, swelling, or discharge. If any of these occur, seek medical attention.

Assessing Severity

In addition to identifying the type of bleeding, it's essential to assess the severity of the injury. Look for the amount of blood loss and the overall condition of the injured person. If a person is losing a lot of blood quickly, showing signs of shock, or has a deep wound, it's critical to get them medical help as soon as possible. Even if the bleeding appears minor, if the person feels faint, confused, or weak, it's best to err on the side of caution and call for emergency assistance.

As you prepare for any potential injuries, remember these extra tips: Always keep a first aid kit handy with sterile dressings, bandages, and antiseptic wipes. Practice applying pressure and bandaging techniques regularly so you feel confident during an emergency. Lastly, consider taking a first aid course to gain hands-on experience and deepen your understanding of bleeding management. Being prepared can help you act effectively when it matters most.

How to Stop Bleeding and Bandage Wounds

When it comes to first aid, knowing how to stop bleeding and bandage wounds is vital. Whether you're at home, outdoors, or in a public place, accidents can happen, and being prepared can make a significant difference in someone's recovery. Quick and effective action can not only prevent excessive blood loss but also reduce the risk of infection and promote healing. In this section, you will learn essential techniques to control bleeding and apply bandages properly, ensuring you can respond effectively in an emergency.

To start, it's important to assess the situation. First, ensure that you and the injured person are safe from any further harm. If the injury is severe, calling for professional medical help is crucial. While waiting for assistance, you can take steps to manage the bleeding.

The first method to stop bleeding involves direct pressure. This technique is effective for most types of wounds. Here's how to do it:

1. Find a Clean Cloth or Bandage: Use a clean cloth, sterile gauze, or even a T-shirt if necessary. Avoid using anything that might cause infection, like dirty or used materials.

2. Apply Direct Pressure: Place the cloth directly over the wound. Use your hand to apply firm, steady pressure. Hold the pressure for at least five to ten minutes without lifting the cloth to check if the bleeding has stopped. Lifting it too soon can disrupt clotting.

3. If Bleeding Persists: If blood soaks through the cloth, do not remove it. Instead, add another layer on top. Continue applying pressure. This method allows the blood to clot and helps minimize blood loss.

In case the direct pressure method does not work and the bleeding is severe, you might need to consider using a tourniquet. A tourniquet is generally used for serious injuries, especially when the bleeding is life-threatening, such as with a limb. Here's how to apply one correctly:

4. Gather Materials: If you have a commercial tourniquet, use it. If not, a belt, cloth strip, or any sturdy material can work. Ensure it is at least two inches wide.

5. Place the Tourniquet above the Injury: Position the tourniquet around the limb, approximately two inches above the wound. Ensure it is not directly over a joint.

6. Tighten the Tourniquet: Twist the tourniquet until the bleeding stops. You should be able to feel the pressure, but it shouldn't cause extreme pain. Once the bleeding has stopped, secure it in place.

7. Note the Time: It's essential to note the time you applied the tourniquet, as prolonged use can lead to tissue damage. Medical professionals need this information to provide appropriate care.

After addressing the bleeding, the next step is to properly bandage the wound. Bandaging helps protect the wound from dirt and bacteria, minimizing the risk of infection. Here's a step-by-step guide to bandaging:

8. Clean the Wound: If the wound is minor and bleeding has stopped, rinse it gently under clean, running water to remove any debris. Avoid using alcohol or hydrogen peroxide, as these can irritate the tissue.

9. Apply an Antibiotic Ointment: After cleaning, apply a thin layer of antibiotic ointment if available. This can help prevent infection.

10. Choose the Right Bandage: Depending on the wound size, select a suitable bandage. For smaller cuts, adhesive bandages (band-aids) are often sufficient. For larger wounds, sterile gauze pads and medical tape work best.

11. Cover the Wound: Place the bandage or gauze pad over the wound, ensuring it is entirely covered. For gauze pads, use medical tape to secure it in place. Be careful not to wrap the tape too tightly, as this can restrict blood flow.

12. Monitor the Wound: Regularly check the bandaged area for signs of infection, which can include increased redness, swelling, or discharge. If any of these signs occur, seek medical attention promptly.

13. Change the Bandage: Change the bandage at least once a day or whenever it becomes wet or dirty. Always wash your hands before changing the bandage to prevent introducing bacteria.

It's also essential to educate yourself about specific types of wounds. For example, puncture wounds, such as those from a nail, require careful monitoring for infection. While they may bleed less, they can trap dirt and bacteria inside, necessitating a doctor's visit.

Additionally, for lacerations or deep cuts, it's best to avoid using adhesive bandages and instead use gauze pads that can absorb more blood and keep the wound protected. In the case of amputations, apply pressure to the stump and elevate it if possible. This helps control bleeding until professional help arrives.

Final Tip

Consider taking a first aid course to enhance your skills and knowledge. Understanding these basic first aid techniques can empower you to respond confidently and effectively in emergencies. Always keep a well-stocked first aid kit on hand and familiarize yourself with its contents, ensuring you're ready to assist in any situation.

Treating Special Wounds: Punctures, Lacerations, and Amputations

When accidents happen, knowing how to treat special wounds like punctures, lacerations, and amputations can be crucial for preserving health and preventing further injury. These types of wounds can vary in severity, and your response can make a significant difference in the outcome. In this section, you'll learn how to recognize these wounds and the essential steps to take for effective treatment.

Punctures

Puncture wounds occur when a sharp object penetrates the skin, creating a small but deep wound. Common causes include nails, needles, and animal bites. While they may appear minor, puncture wounds can lead to serious infections, especially if they are not cleaned properly.

If you encounter someone with a puncture wound, first assess the situation to determine the severity of the injury. If the object is still embedded in the wound, do not remove it, as this could cause further bleeding or damage. Instead, stabilize the object with sterile gauze or cloth to minimize movement.

Next, clean the area around the puncture with soap and water. Avoid using alcohol or hydrogen peroxide directly on the wound, as these can irritate the tissue. Once cleaned, apply an antibiotic ointment to help prevent infection, and cover the wound with a sterile bandage. It's essential to keep an eye on the wound over the next few days for signs of infection, such as increased redness, swelling, or discharge.

If the wound is deep, if the person has not had a tetanus shot in the last five years, or if there are signs of infection, seek professional medical assistance promptly. In some cases, puncture wounds may require stitches or further treatment from a healthcare provider.

Lacerations

Lacerations are cuts in the skin that can vary widely in depth and severity. They can be caused by sharp objects, falls, or even animal bites. Unlike punctures, lacerations tend to bleed more and may require specific attention based on their severity.

To treat a laceration, start by applying direct pressure to stop any bleeding. Use a clean cloth or sterile gauze, applying firm pressure for about 10 minutes. If the bleeding does not stop, maintain pressure and seek medical help. If the bleeding does subside, gently clean the wound with soap and water, being careful not to scrub the area, which can worsen the injury.

Once cleaned, assess the laceration to determine if stitches are necessary. If the edges of the cut are jagged or if the wound is deeper than half an inch, it's best to consult a medical professional for stitches or adhesive strips to close the wound. For smaller lacerations, you can apply an antibiotic ointment and cover it with a sterile bandage.

Keep the laceration clean and change the bandage daily or if it becomes wet or dirty. Watch for signs of infection, and if you notice increasing pain, swelling, or discharge, seek medical attention.

Amputations

An amputation is a severe injury where a part of the body is severed, either completely or partially. This type of injury can be life-threatening and requires immediate action. If someone experiences an amputation, the priority is to control the bleeding and preserve the severed part for potential reattachment.

Begin by calling emergency services immediately. While waiting for help, apply direct pressure to the wound using a clean cloth or sterile bandage. If the bleeding is severe, you may need to apply a tourniquet above the injury site. Use a cloth or bandage to create a tight wrap around the limb, but do not cut off circulation completely.

To preserve the amputated part, rinse it gently with saline or clean water if available. Wrap it in a clean cloth or sterile gauze, then place it in a waterproof bag or container. Keep the severed part cool, but do not place it directly on ice. Instead, place the container with the amputated part in a bowl of ice water. This will help preserve it until medical professionals can assess the injury.

Amputation injuries require specialized medical treatment. Once you have controlled the bleeding and preserved the severed part, monitor the person for shock, which can occur due to severe blood loss. Signs of shock include weakness, confusion, rapid breathing, and a weak pulse. If you notice these symptoms, lay the person down, elevate their legs, and keep them warm until help arrives.

Treating special wounds like punctures, lacerations, and amputations requires knowledge and a calm approach. Always prioritize safety by wearing gloves if available and keeping the injured person as calm as possible. Monitor for signs of infection and other complications, and do not hesitate to seek medical help when necessary.

Extra Tips

1. First Aid Kit: Keep a well-stocked first aid kit at home and in your car. Make sure it includes adhesive bandages, antiseptic wipes, gauze, and antibiotic ointment.

2. Tetanus Vaccination: Ensure that you and your family members are up to date on tetanus vaccinations, especially if you frequently engage in activities that might cause cuts or punctures.

3. Education: Consider taking a first aid and CPR course to enhance your skills and confidence in handling emergencies effectively.

By being prepared and informed, you can respond quickly and effectively to special wounds, potentially saving a life or preventing further injury.

Chapter 5: Fractures, Sprains, and Dislocations

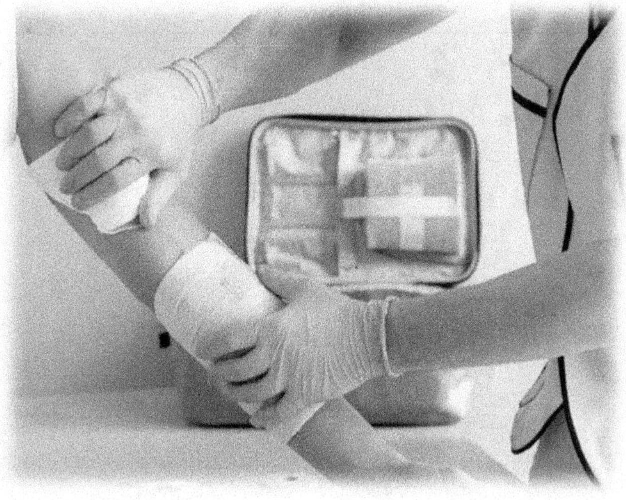

During a ski trip, Lora's friend, Mike, took a bad fall and severely injured his ankle. Lora quickly assessed the damage, recognizing the signs of a sprain. She immobilized Mike's ankle using a makeshift splint and applied ice to reduce swelling. Then, she carefully assisted Mike down the mountain to seek medical attention. Thanks to Lora's swift and knowledgeable care, Mike avoided further injury and made a full recovery. Her expertise demonstrated the importance of proper fracture, sprain, and dislocation management in preventing long-term damage and promoting optimal healing.

Recognizing and Immobilizing Fractures

When it comes to dealing with injuries, knowing how to recognize and immobilize fractures is essential. Fractures, or broken bones, can happen unexpectedly, and understanding their signs and the correct way to manage them can make a significant difference in the outcome for the injured person. This guide will walk you through identifying fractures and the necessary steps to immobilize them safely.

Recognizing a fracture is the first critical step in providing first aid. There are several signs that indicate a bone may be broken. Look for swelling or bruising around the injury site, which is common. The person may also report pain, especially when trying to move the affected area. If you see an abnormal angle or a bone protruding through the skin, it is essential to seek help immediately, as this is a clear indication of a severe fracture.

You might also notice that the injured person has difficulty moving the limb or is reluctant to use it at all. These symptoms can indicate a fracture, sprain, or strain, but in any case, it's important to proceed with caution. If you suspect a fracture, avoid moving the person or the injured limb unnecessarily, as this could cause further injury.

When assessing the injury, try to keep the person calm. Reassure them that help is on the way and encourage them to remain still. If the injury is on a limb, ask them to keep it elevated if possible. This can help reduce swelling and pain while waiting for professional medical assistance.

Once you suspect a fracture, the next step is immobilization. Immobilizing the fracture is crucial to prevent further injury and to alleviate pain. You can use a variety of materials to create a splint. The goal is to hold the broken bone in place so it doesn't move, which can reduce the risk of further damage to the surrounding tissues and blood vessels.

To immobilize a fracture, you'll need a few basic materials. If you have access to a commercial splint, that's great! However, if you don't, you can use any sturdy object like a rolled-up magazine, a piece of cardboard, or even a stick. You'll want something that can provide stability to the injured limb. The splint should extend beyond the fracture site to secure both the joint above and below the fracture.

Start by carefully aligning the injured limb in its natural position. If the limb is bent at an odd angle, do not attempt to realign it. Instead, secure it in the position it is currently in. Use padding if available—such as towels, clothing, or other soft materials—around the fracture site to make the splint more comfortable. This padding will help absorb any shocks or pressure during movement.

Once you have the splint ready, place it alongside the injured limb and use adhesive tape, gauze, or cloth strips to secure the splint in place. Make sure not to wrap it too tightly, as this could restrict blood flow. You should be able to slide one or two fingers under the bandage comfortably. Check the fingers or toes of the injured limb for circulation by observing their color and temperature. They should remain warm and pink. If they become pale or cold, loosen the wrap immediately.

After immobilizing the fracture, you should ensure that the injured person is comfortable. Offer them reassurance and check for any signs of shock, which can include pale skin, rapid breathing, or confusion. If you notice any of these symptoms, lay the person down and elevate their legs if possible. Keep them warm with a blanket or jacket until professional help arrives.

While waiting for emergency services, encourage the injured person to remain as still as possible. Keep an eye on their condition and be ready to provide further assistance if their situation changes. It's also a good idea to avoid giving them anything to eat or drink, as they may require surgery or other medical procedures once help arrives.

Understanding how to recognize and immobilize fractures can be invaluable in emergency situations. Being prepared with the right knowledge can make a significant difference in ensuring the best possible outcome for someone with a suspected fracture.

Extra Tips:

Always seek professional medical help for any suspected fractures, especially if there is deformity or if the injury is severe. Practicing these skills in a first aid course can also enhance your confidence and readiness to respond in real-life situations. Remember, the quicker you act and stabilize the injury, the better the chances of a smooth recovery.

Managing Sprains and Strains

When it comes to managing sprains and strains, knowing how to respond quickly and effectively can make a significant difference in recovery time and overall healing. Sprains and strains are common injuries, especially for those who lead active lifestyles or participate in sports. Understanding how to identify and treat these injuries can help you provide proper care and alleviate pain.

A sprain occurs when ligaments—the strong bands of tissue that connect bones at a joint—are stretched or torn. This often happens during activities that involve sudden twists, falls, or impacts. On the other hand, a strain involves muscles or tendons, which are the tissues that connect muscles to bones. Strains occur when these muscles or tendons are overstretched or torn, often as a result of lifting heavy objects, twisting, or excessive force. Both types of injuries can cause pain, swelling, bruising, and limited movement in the affected area.

Identifying a sprain or strain is the first step in effective management. Look for key symptoms: pain around the joint or muscle, swelling, bruising, and difficulty using the affected area. You might also hear a popping sound at the moment of injury. If you suspect a more severe injury, such as a fracture, it's crucial to seek medical attention.

Once you've assessed the injury, you can implement the R.I.C.E. method, a widely recommended approach for managing sprains and strains. R.I.C.E. stands for Rest, Ice, Compression, and Elevation.

Rest: The first and most important step is to stop using the injured area. This helps prevent further damage. You should avoid any activity that causes pain or discomfort. If it's a leg or foot injury, consider using crutches or a brace to keep weight off the area.

Ice: Apply ice to the injured area as soon as possible after the injury occurs. Ice helps reduce swelling and numbs the pain. Wrap ice in a cloth or use a cold pack and apply it for about 15 to 20 minutes every hour during the first 24 to 48 hours. Avoid placing ice directly on the skin, as this can lead to frostbite.

Compression: Use an elastic bandage or wrap to compress the injured area. This helps reduce swelling and provides support. Ensure that the bandage is snug but not so tight that it cuts off circulation. If you notice increased pain, swelling, or numbness, loosen the bandage.

Elevation: Elevating the injured area helps decrease swelling by allowing fluids to drain away from the site of injury. If it's a sprained ankle, prop your foot on a pillow while sitting or lying down. Try to keep the area elevated above the level of your heart for as long as possible during the first few days.

After the initial treatment, monitor the injury closely. If pain and swelling do not improve within a few days, or if symptoms worsen, seek medical attention. A healthcare provider may recommend further evaluation, such as an X-ray or MRI, to rule out fractures or other serious injuries.

Once you start feeling better, gentle stretching and strengthening exercises can aid in recovery. However, be careful not to push through pain. Gradually reintroduce movement, and avoid activities that may cause a recurrence of the injury until you have fully healed. Physical therapy may also be beneficial if your injury is more severe, as a trained professional can provide targeted exercises to improve strength and flexibility.

For ongoing care, consider over-the-counter pain relievers like ibuprofen or acetaminophen to help manage discomfort. Always follow the instructions on the label and consult with a healthcare professional if you have any concerns or if the pain persists.

Additionally, be aware of your body's signals. Rest is just as important in the recovery phase as it is immediately following the injury.

Rushing back into activity too soon can lead to reinjury or chronic pain.

Extra Tip

As a final tip, consider investing in a first aid kit that includes items specifically for sprains and strains, such as elastic bandages and cold packs. This ensures that you are prepared to handle any minor injuries that may occur during everyday activities or sports. Having the right tools on hand can make it easier to manage these common injuries effectively.

Taking these steps will not only help in managing sprains and strains but will also contribute to better overall health and safety in your daily activities.

First Aid for Dislocations and Joint Injuries

Dislocations and joint injuries can occur during everyday activities, sports, or accidents. Recognizing the signs and knowing how to respond can make a significant difference in managing these injuries effectively. This section will guide you through understanding dislocations and joint injuries, how to assess the situation, and the steps to take for first aid.

Dislocations happen when the ends of bones in a joint are forced out of their normal positions. Common areas for dislocations include the shoulder, elbow, fingers, and kneecap. On the other hand, joint injuries can include sprains and strains, which affect the ligaments and muscles surrounding the joint. Sprains occur when ligaments are stretched or torn, while strains involve muscles or tendons. Understanding the difference between these injuries is crucial for proper first aid treatment.

Recognizing Dislocations and Joint Injuries

The first step in providing effective first aid is recognizing the symptoms of dislocations and joint injuries. A dislocated joint often appears visibly deformed, and the affected area may swell rapidly. You might notice that the person experiences severe pain and an inability to use the joint. In contrast, sprains can present with swelling, bruising, and pain, which may be moderate to severe depending on the injury's extent.

If you suspect a dislocation, assess the area carefully. Look for unusual angles or positions of the joint, and pay attention to any visible swelling or bruising. Encourage the injured person to remain as still as possible, as movement could worsen the injury.

Initial First Aid Steps

Once you identify a dislocation or joint injury, your immediate response is critical. Here's a step-by-step guide to follow:

1. Call for Help: If the injury is severe, such as a dislocation, call for emergency medical assistance immediately. Explain the situation clearly so they can provide the right help.

2. Do Not Attempt to Reposition the Joint: It might be tempting to try and put the joint back in place, but this can cause further damage to the surrounding tissues, nerves, and blood vessels. Always wait for a medical professional to handle the dislocation.

3. Stabilize the Joint: If it's a joint injury, try to immobilize the affected area to prevent any movement. You can use a splint or make one with any rigid material available, such as a rolled-up magazine or a piece of cardboard. For a dislocated shoulder, keep the arm close to the body and support it with a sling if you have one.

4. Apply Ice: To reduce swelling and relieve pain, apply an ice pack wrapped in a cloth to the injured area. Ice should be used for about 15-20 minutes at a time, with breaks in between to avoid frostbite.

5. Monitor for Shock: Keep an eye on the injured person for signs of shock, which may include pale skin, rapid breathing, and confusion. If you suspect they are going into shock, keep them lying down, elevate their legs if it's safe, and reassure them until help arrives.

When to Seek Medical Attention

Even if the injury seems minor, it's essential to seek medical attention after providing initial first aid. A healthcare professional will evaluate the injury more thoroughly, conduct necessary imaging, and determine the appropriate treatment. In cases of severe dislocations or joint injuries, surgery may be needed to restore normal function.

Managing Pain and Recovery

Once medical help has been provided, managing pain is crucial for recovery. Over-the-counter pain relievers, such as ibuprofen or acetaminophen, can help reduce discomfort. However, it's important to follow the dosage instructions on the label or as advised by a healthcare professional.

During recovery, the affected joint may require rest and protection. Depending on the severity of the injury, your healthcare provider may recommend physical therapy to restore strength and mobility. Always follow their guidance for rehabilitation exercises and activity restrictions.

Extra Tip

Understanding how to recognize and respond to dislocations and joint injuries is vital for effective first aid. Always prioritize safety and seek professional help when needed. Here are a few extra tips: Keep a first aid kit stocked with splints and ice packs, educate family members on how to respond to joint injuries, and consider taking a first aid course to enhance your skills. Being prepared can make a significant difference in an emergency.

Chapter 6: Burns and Scalds

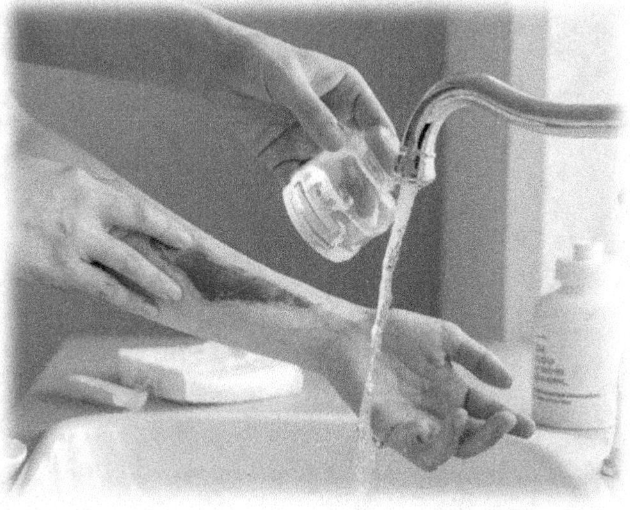

While camping, Fiona's son accidentally spilled boiling water on his arm. Fiona swiftly responded, cooling the burn with cool water for 10 minutes and removing nearby clothing and jewelry. She then applied a sterile dressing and gave her son pain relief medication. Recognizing the severity of the burn, Fiona sought immediate medical attention. Thanks to Fiona's prompt and proper care, her son's burn healed quickly with minimal scarring. Her calm and effective response demonstrated the importance of knowing burn and scald treatment protocols.

Understanding the Different Degrees of Burns

Burns are injuries that occur when your skin or body tissues come into contact with heat, chemicals, electricity, or radiation. Understanding the different degrees of burns is crucial because it helps you assess the severity of the injury and determine the appropriate first aid treatment. This knowledge can be life-saving and may prevent further complications.

Burns are classified into three main degrees: first-degree, second-degree, and third-degree. Each degree reflects the severity of the burn and the layers of skin that are affected. Let's explore each type of burn in detail, including how to recognize them and the best way to respond.

First-Degree Burns

First-degree burns are the mildest form of burn and primarily affect the outer layer of skin, known as the epidermis. These burns are usually caused by brief contact with a hot object, sun exposure, or mild chemical exposure. You can recognize a first-degree burn by the following characteristics:

- **Redness**: The affected area will appear red and may be slightly swollen.

- **Pain**: You will likely experience pain in the burn area, which can range from mild to moderate.

- **Dryness**: The skin will feel dry and may be sensitive to touch.

When treating a first-degree burn, the main goal is to relieve pain and promote healing. Here are some practical steps to follow:

1. **Cool the Burn**: As soon as you realize you have a first-degree burn, run cool (not cold) water over the affected area for about 10 to 20 minutes. If running water isn't available, you can apply a clean, cool, damp cloth to the burn.

2. **Avoid Ice:** Do not apply ice directly to the burn, as it can cause further damage to the skin.

3. Pain Relief: Over-the-counter pain relievers, such as ibuprofen or acetaminophen, can help manage pain and reduce inflammation.

4. Moisturize: After cooling the burn, apply a gentle moisturizer or aloe vera gel to soothe the skin. Avoid products with alcohol, which can irritate the burn.

5. Cover the Area: If needed, cover the burn with a sterile bandage or a non-stick dressing to protect it from dirt and further irritation.

First-degree burns typically heal within three to six days without medical intervention. Keep an eye on the burn for signs of infection, such as increased redness, swelling, or pus.

Second-Degree Burns

Second-degree burns are more severe and affect both the epidermis and the second layer of skin, known as the dermis. These burns can occur from prolonged exposure to hot liquids, flames, or severe sunburn. You can identify a second-degree burn by these features:

- **Blisters**: The skin may form blisters filled with clear fluid.

- **Intense Pain**: These burns are often more painful than first-degree burns.

- **Swelling**: The area around the burn may be swollen and red.

Second-degree burns require more careful treatment. Here's how to manage them effectively:

1. **Cool the Burn:** Just like with first-degree burns, cool the affected area immediately by running it under cool water for about 10 to 20 minutes. This helps reduce pain and inflammation.

2. **Do Not Break Blisters**: If blisters form, do not pop them, as this can lead to infection. If blisters break on their own, gently wash the area with soap and water and apply a clean dressing.

3. **Use Pain Relievers**: Over-the-counter pain medications can help manage discomfort.

Follow the recommended dosages on the packaging.

4. Moisturize: After cooling the burn, apply a moisturizing lotion or aloe vera gel. Keep the area clean and moisturized to promote healing.

5. Cover the Burn: Use a non-stick bandage or sterile dressing to cover the burn and protect it from infection. Change the dressing daily or if it becomes wet or dirty.

Healing time for second-degree burns varies, but they typically take two to three weeks to heal. If you notice signs of infection or if the burn covers a large area, seek medical attention.

Third-Degree Burns

Third-degree burns are the most severe type, affecting all layers of the skin and potentially damaging underlying tissues, including muscle and bone. These burns can result from contact with flames, scalding liquids, or electrical injuries. Signs of a third-degree burn include:

- **White or Charred Skin**: The affected area may appear white, leathery, or charred.

- **Lack of Pain**: Surprisingly, third-degree burns may not be painful at the burn site due to nerve damage.

- **Severe Swelling**: The area may be swollen and may develop blisters.

Third-degree burns require immediate medical attention. Do not attempt to treat these burns at home. Instead, follow these steps while waiting for emergency services:

1. **Call for Help:** Dial emergency services right away if you suspect a third-degree burn.

2. **Prevent Shock**: Lay the person flat, if possible, and cover them with a clean, dry blanket to prevent shock.

3. **Do Not Immerse in Water**: Avoid soaking a third-degree burn in water, as this can lead to further injury.

4. Do Not Remove Burned Clothing: If clothing is stuck to the burn, do not attempt to remove it. Instead, cover the area with a clean cloth or dressing.

5. Monitor Vital Signs: Keep an eye on the person's breathing and consciousness until help arrives.

Healing from a third-degree burn can take a long time and often requires medical treatment, including surgery and rehabilitation.

Understanding the degrees of burns and how to respond can make a significant difference in the outcome of burn injuries. By knowing how to assess and treat burns, you can help ensure a faster recovery and minimize complications.

Extra Tips:

Always keep a first aid kit handy, including burn ointments and dressings. If you're spending time outdoors, apply sunscreen regularly to protect against sunburn. Remember that for any burn that appears severe, covers a large area, or is on the face, hands, feet, or genitals, professional medical treatment is essential.

Immediate Treatment for Burns and Scalds

Burns and scalds are common injuries that can happen to anyone, from children to adults. Knowing how to treat these injuries promptly and correctly is crucial in minimizing damage to the skin and preventing complications. Burns can result from various sources, including heat, chemicals, electricity, and radiation, while scalds are specifically caused by hot liquids or steam. Immediate and appropriate treatment can make a significant difference in healing and recovery.

When a burn or scald occurs, your first step is to ensure the safety of everyone involved. If the injury is due to a fire or electrical source, turn off the source of the heat if it's safe to do so. For scalds, remove the person from the hot liquid or steam source immediately. Assess the situation before proceeding with treatment, as understanding the severity of the injury will guide your next steps.

The first principle in treating burns and scalds is to cool the affected area. Quickly running cool (not cold) water over the burn is one of the most effective ways to reduce the temperature of the skin and alleviate pain. Aim to do this within the first 20 minutes after the injury, as this is when it can be most beneficial. You should keep the area under cool water for at least 10 to 20 minutes, as this helps stop the burning process and can lessen tissue damage.

If running water isn't available, you can use a cool, wet compress instead. Just make sure it's clean to prevent infection. Avoid using ice or very cold water, as these can cause further damage to the skin and worsen the injury. It's essential to be gentle during this cooling process, as rough handling can lead to more harm.

After cooling the burn, assess its severity. Burns are generally categorized into three degrees:

1. First-degree burns affect only the outer layer of skin, causing redness and mild pain. These can usually be treated at home.

2. Second-degree burns penetrate deeper, affecting both the outer layer and the layer beneath it. They cause redness, swelling, and blistering. These burns may require medical attention, especially if they cover a large area.

3. Third-degree burns damage all layers of the skin and can involve deeper tissues. The area may appear white, charred, or leathery, and can be painless due to nerve damage. These burns always require immediate medical assistance.

Once you have assessed the severity of the burn, it's time to clean the area. Use mild soap and water to gently cleanse the burn, ensuring you don't break any blisters that may have formed. Blisters act as a protective barrier against infection, so it's important to leave them intact if possible. After cleaning, gently pat the area dry with a clean cloth.

If the burn is mild (first-degree or small second-degree), you can apply a sterile, non-adhesive dressing to protect the area from dirt and friction. Do not use cotton balls or fluffy dressings, as these can stick to the burn and cause pain when removed. For second-degree burns, you may also apply a topical antibiotic ointment to help prevent infection.

For pain relief, over-the-counter medications such as ibuprofen or acetaminophen can be helpful. Always follow the dosing instructions on the packaging, and consult with a healthcare professional if you're unsure. If the burn covers a large area or if it's on the face, hands, feet, or genitals, seek medical attention promptly, as these areas are more sensitive and can result in complications.

In the case of chemical burns, the first step is to remove the person from the source of the chemical. Rinse the area with cool water for at least 20 minutes, as this helps to dilute and wash away the chemical. It's vital to seek medical help for chemical burns, as specific treatments may be necessary based on the type of chemical involved.

Electrical burns can be more complicated due to the potential for internal injuries. If someone has been injured by electricity, it's crucial to avoid touching them until the power source has been turned off. Call emergency services immediately, as they will need to assess for internal injuries even if the external injuries appear minor.

Lastly, monitor the affected person for signs of infection, especially in the days following the injury. Symptoms of infection can include increased redness, swelling, pus, or fever. If any of these signs occur, seek medical attention promptly.

Extra Tips:

Always keep a first-aid kit handy that includes burn dressings and topical ointments. It's also helpful to familiarize yourself with the local emergency services and have their contact information accessible. Educate children about the dangers of hot surfaces, liquids, and flames to prevent burns before they happen. Taking these precautions can greatly enhance your preparedness for dealing with burns and scalds effectively.

Long-Term Care and Recovery for Burn Victims

Long-term care and recovery for burn victims is a critical aspect of the healing process. After the initial treatment of burns, whether from heat, chemicals, or electricity, it's essential to understand how to support a burn victim's ongoing recovery. Proper care can help minimize scarring, promote healing, and restore the individual's quality of life.

Burn recovery can take a long time, and it's important to approach it with patience and understanding. Depending on the severity of the burn, a victim may experience physical, emotional, and psychological challenges. Understanding these aspects is key to providing effective support.

To start, it's essential to recognize that burns are classified into three degrees: first-degree burns affect only the outer layer of skin, second-degree burns impact the outer layer and part of the underlying layer, and third-degree burns damage deeper tissues. The treatment approach and recovery process vary significantly based on the degree of the burn.

Wound Care

After initial treatment, regular wound care is crucial for promoting healing and preventing infection. For first-degree burns, keep the area clean and apply soothing lotions like aloe vera to keep the skin hydrated. For second-degree burns, follow your healthcare provider's instructions regarding dressings. These burns require more care, as blisters can form. Always avoid popping blisters, as this can lead to infections. Instead, cover the area with a sterile, non-stick bandage and change it regularly to keep the wound clean.

In the case of third-degree burns, professional medical treatment is often necessary, which may include skin grafts. During recovery, it's important to follow your healthcare team's guidance closely. This may include caring for grafted areas and keeping them clean. Always watch for signs of infection, such as increased redness, swelling, or discharge from the wound.

Managing Pain and Discomfort

Pain management is an important part of recovery. Depending on the severity of the burn, victims may experience pain that requires medication. Over-the-counter pain relievers like acetaminophen or ibuprofen can be effective for milder pain. However, always consult with a healthcare professional for more severe pain, as they may prescribe stronger medications.

As part of long-term care, encourage the victim to participate in gentle stretching exercises to maintain mobility. Scar tissue can limit movement, especially with more serious burns, so it's important to keep the affected area flexible. Gentle stretching, along with physical therapy, can help improve mobility and reduce stiffness.

Nutrition and Hydration

Good nutrition is vital for recovery. The body needs energy and nutrients to heal, so encourage the burn victim to consume a balanced diet rich in proteins, vitamins, and minerals. Proteins play a crucial role in repairing tissues, while vitamins A and C can support skin health and immune function. Foods like lean meats, fish, eggs, dairy, fruits, and vegetables are all beneficial.

Staying hydrated is also important, as burns can lead to fluid loss. Ensure the victim drinks plenty of water throughout the day. Hydration helps support the healing process and keeps the skin moist.

Emotional Support

Long-term recovery from burns is not just physical; emotional support is equally important. Many burn victims may experience anxiety, depression, or post-traumatic stress disorder (PTSD) related to their injury. Open communication is key. Encourage the victim to talk about their feelings and experiences. Be a good listener and validate their emotions.

In some cases, professional counseling may be beneficial. Support groups specifically for burn victims can also provide a sense of community and understanding. Connecting with others who have faced similar experiences can be incredibly healing.

Preventing Scarring

After healing, scars may remain, especially with deeper burns. To minimize scarring, it's crucial to follow the advice of healthcare professionals. They may recommend silicone gel sheets or other topical treatments to reduce scar formation. Keeping scars moisturized and protected from the sun can also help them heal better.

Physical therapy can play a significant role in scar management. Specialized exercises can help improve the appearance of scars and prevent contractures, which is when the skin becomes tight and limits movement.

Regular Follow-Ups

Long-term care for burn victims includes regular follow-up appointments with healthcare providers. These visits allow for monitoring the healing process and addressing any complications early. During these check-ups, healthcare professionals can assess the burn area and provide further guidance on care and recovery.

Extra Tip

The long-term care and recovery of burn victims involve a multi-faceted approach that includes wound care, pain management, nutrition, emotional support, and regular follow-ups. By following these guidelines, caregivers can help burn victims navigate the recovery process more effectively. Remember, every individual's healing journey is unique, so it's important to remain patient and supportive throughout their recovery.

Chapter 7: Choking and Airway Obstructions

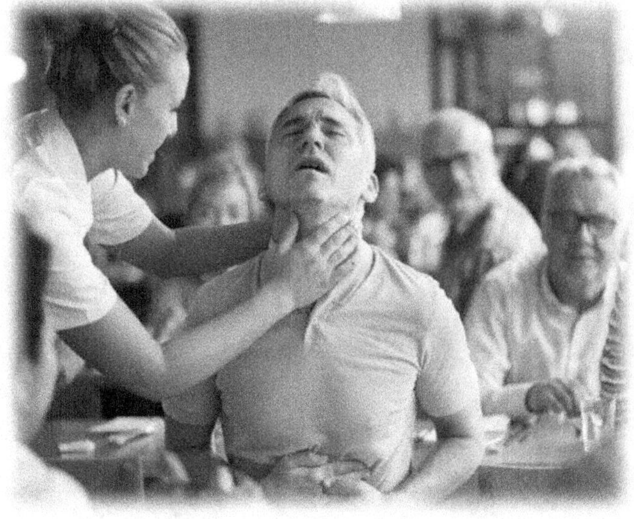

Tragedy struck when 3-year-old Emma began choking on a grape at a family gathering. Her aunt, panicked and unaware of proper first aid, attempted to pat Emma's back instead of performing the Heimlich maneuver. Precious minutes ticked by as Emma's airway remained blocked. By the time paramedics arrived, irreversible brain damage had occurred, leaving

Emma with lifelong disabilities. This heartbreaking incident highlights the devastating consequences of inadequate training in choking and airway obstruction response. Knowing the proper techniques can mean the difference between life and death.

Recognizing Signs of Choking

Choking is a life-threatening emergency that can happen in seconds, especially when food or small objects block the airway. Knowing how to recognize the signs of choking can mean the difference between life and death. Whether you're caring for an adult, child, or infant, understanding these signals is crucial so that you can act quickly.

When someone is choking, their airway is either fully or partially obstructed. Depending on the severity, their reactions can vary, so it's important to be able to differentiate between mild and severe choking. This helps you provide the right care and avoid unnecessary panic.

The signs of choking are often sudden and noticeable. In many cases, the person will immediately place their hands on their throat—a universal sign of choking. However, this is not always the case, especially in younger children or infants. You need to be observant of other signals that may indicate someone is having trouble breathing due to a blocked airway.

1. Coughing and Gagging

When the airway is only partially blocked, the person may still be able to cough, gag, or make wheezing sounds. Coughing is often the body's natural response to try and clear the obstruction. You might hear the individual coughing forcefully or even see them attempt to gag the item out of their throat. While this is still a dangerous situation, a strong cough means there is some air getting through. You should encourage them to keep coughing, as this might help dislodge the object on its own.

2. Inability to Speak or Make Noise

If someone is choking severely, they may not be able to speak or make any sound. This is a major red flag. A fully blocked airway means that no air is passing through the vocal cords, which makes it impossible for the person to talk. If they open their mouth as if to speak or cry but nothing comes out, you must act immediately to help them.

3. Breathing Difficulties

Pay close attention to breathing patterns. In severe cases of choking, the individual may not be able to breathe at all, or they may take very weak, gasping breaths. You might notice their chest rising but little to no airflow. Without oxygen, the person's lips and face may start turning blue or gray, which is a sign of cyanosis—a dangerous condition where the body isn't getting enough oxygen.

4. Silent Choking in Children and Infants

Infants and young children may not be able to communicate their distress as clearly as adults can. Silent choking is especially common among babies. Instead of coughing or gagging, they might simply stop breathing altogether. Watch for sudden stillness, wide eyes, or a look of panic. If a baby suddenly becomes unusually quiet or their face begins to change color, check their airway immediately.

5. Clutching the Throat

One of the most well-known signs of choking is someone clutching their throat with one or both hands. This is often referred to as the "universal choking sign." When people are unable to speak or breathe properly, their first instinct is to grab their neck in a desperate attempt to clear the airway. If you see someone making this gesture, it's a clear signal that they need help.

6. Loss of Consciousness

If the blockage isn't cleared quickly, choking can lead to loss of consciousness. When the brain is deprived of oxygen for too long, it will start shutting down, and the person may faint. If this happens, you'll need to perform CPR immediately, as the person is at risk of brain damage or death.

7. High-Pitched Sounds or No Sound at All

During a severe choking episode, the airway may be partially or completely obstructed. If it's partially blocked, you might hear a high-pitched whistling noise as the person tries to breathe. If it's fully blocked, there may be no sound at all. Any time you hear or see these signs, it's an indication that the airway is compromised and immediate intervention is required.

8. Distress and Panic

Choking victims often display signs of intense distress and panic. They may become agitated, restless, and fearful as they struggle for air. It's important for you to stay calm in this situation so you can think clearly and take appropriate steps to help them. If the person starts thrashing or appears frantic, you'll need to act quickly to perform first aid measures.

9. Color Changes in Skin Tone

The skin, particularly around the lips, face, and fingertips, may change color due to lack of oxygen. This is one of the more serious signs that the airway is fully blocked. If the person's skin starts to turn blue, purple, or gray, it means the body is not receiving enough oxygen, and you should respond immediately.

Extra Tips

When it comes to recognizing choking, time is of the essence. Always observe the person's body language and listen to their breathing. The faster you notice the signs, the quicker you can respond with appropriate first aid techniques, such as back blows or abdominal thrusts. Tip: Keep in mind that choking in babies requires different techniques, like gentle back blows and chest thrusts, as their bodies are more delicate.

First Aid for Choking in Adults, Children, and Infants

When someone is choking, time is critical. Knowing how to provide first aid for choking can be the difference between life and death. It's important to understand that the approach for dealing with choking differs based on the age of the person. Choking in adults, children, and infants requires different methods of intervention, but the goal remains the same: to clear the airway and restore normal breathing as quickly as possible. Let's explore the practical steps you should follow in each scenario, focusing on how to respond effectively and calmly.

Understanding Choking and Its Risks

Choking occurs when an object—usually food—gets stuck in the throat or windpipe, blocking airflow. A person who is choking may not be able to breathe or speak. The inability to get oxygen to the lungs causes rapid distress, and if the blockage isn't removed, it can lead to unconsciousness and even death. While choking can happen to anyone, it's particularly common in young children who tend to put small objects or large pieces of food into their mouths and in older adults who might have difficulty swallowing.

The key signs of choking include:

- The person clutching their throat

- Inability to speak or breathe

- Panic or distress

- Redness or bluish skin tone

- Wheezing or coughing weakly

First Aid for Adults and Older Children (Ages 8+)

When an adult or older child is choking, you need to act fast but stay calm. If the person is coughing, encourage them to continue, as this means their airway is only partially blocked, and they may be able to dislodge the object on their own.

1. Check if they can cough or breathe: If they cannot make any noise and are struggling to breathe, it's time to take action. Ask them if they are choking, and if they nod or cannot respond, proceed with the following steps.

2. Back Blows: Stand slightly behind the person and to the side. Support their chest with one hand and use the heel of your other hand to deliver five firm back blows between the shoulder blades. The force of the blows is intended to dislodge the object causing the blockage.

3. Abdominal Thrusts (Heimlich maneuver): If the back blows do not work, perform abdominal thrusts. Stand behind the person, wrap your arms around their waist, and make a fist with one hand. Place the thumb side of your fist just above their belly button. Grasp your fist with your other hand and press inward and upward with quick, forceful movements.

Perform up to five abdominal thrusts, checking after each one to see if the blockage has been cleared.

4. Repeat if Necessary: Alternate between five back blows and five abdominal thrusts until the object is expelled or the person becomes unresponsive. If they become unconscious, you'll need to begin CPR (cardiopulmonary resuscitation) and call for emergency help.

First Aid for Children (Ages 1 to 8)

The procedure for helping a choking child is very similar to that of an adult, but with a few adjustments due to their smaller size. First, ensure you are supporting their head and body carefully, as children are more fragile than adults.

1. Encourage Coughing: If the child is still able to cough, encourage them to keep coughing to try and expel the object on their own.

2. Back Blows and Abdominal Thrusts: Just as with an adult, if the child cannot cough, breathe, or speak, begin with five back blows, followed by five abdominal thrusts. For younger children, it's important to be gentle yet firm. Use less force than you would with an adult, but still aim to dislodge the object. Kneel down or stand behind them, wrapping your arms around their waist, and apply upward pressure.

3. Monitor Closely: Children may panic more quickly than adults, so be sure to reassure them throughout the process. If they become unconscious, start CPR immediately.

First Aid for Infants (Under 1 Year Old)

Choking in infants is particularly dangerous since their airways are so small, and they are unable to effectively cough or clear the airway on their own. The first aid procedure for infants differs greatly from adults and children.

1. Lay the Infant Face Down: Position the infant face down on your forearm, supporting their head and neck with your hand. Ensure that the infant's head is lower than their body. Rest your forearm on your thigh to provide stability.

2. Give Back Blows: Using the heel of your hand, give up to five gentle but firm back blows between the infant's shoulder blades. Be sure to apply enough pressure to dislodge the object, but don't use too much force, as their bodies are delicate.

3. Chest Thrusts: If the object isn't expelled after the back blows, turn the infant onto their back, resting them on your thigh. Use two fingers to perform up to five quick chest thrusts in the center of their chest, just below the nipple line. Push down about 1.5 inches with each thrust. The goal is to force the object out by increasing pressure in the chest.

4. Repeat if Necessary: Continue alternating between back blows and chest thrusts until the object is dislodged or the infant becomes unconscious. If the infant becomes unresponsive, start infant CPR immediately and call for emergency assistance.

Extra Tips for Preventing Choking

In addition to knowing how to provide first aid for choking, it's important to take steps to prevent choking incidents. For adults and older children, encourage small bites, chew food thoroughly, and avoid talking or laughing while eating. For younger children and infants, cut food into small pieces, avoid giving them round or hard foods (such as grapes, nuts, or candy), and keep small objects out of reach.

For infants, always supervise them during meals and be aware of common choking hazards in their environment. Prevention is always better than cure, but having this knowledge can ensure you're prepared if an emergency arises.

When to Perform Back Blows and Abdominal Thrusts

Choking is a frightening and potentially life-threatening emergency that can happen to anyone, regardless of age. Knowing when and how to act during a choking incident is vital in first aid. One of the key actions you can take is using back blows and abdominal thrusts (also known as the Heimlich maneuver) to help dislodge the object causing the blockage. However, it's important to understand when each technique is appropriate and how to perform them safely to avoid causing further injury.

When a person chokes, their airway becomes blocked, preventing air from reaching their lungs. If this happens, they may not be able to cough or breathe properly. If the airway is only partially blocked, the person might still be able to cough, and you should encourage them to do so. But if the choking is severe and the person is struggling to breathe, immediate action is necessary. That's when back blows and abdominal thrusts come into play.

Recognizing Severe Choking

The first step is to recognize the signs of severe choking. If the person cannot cough, speak, or breathe, and is showing signs of distress such as clutching their throat, turning blue, or panicking, this indicates a completely blocked airway. You must act quickly. Severe choking may result from food, small objects, or even fluids that have gone down the wrong way, especially in children. The key here is to stay calm and start by trying back blows.

How to Perform Back Blows

Back blows are typically the first step in helping someone who is choking. They are most effective when the object is high up in the airway. To perform back blows:

1. Stand behind the person, slightly to one side.

2. Support their chest with one hand to ensure they do not fall forward.

3. With the heel of your other hand, deliver a firm blow between their shoulder blades. The purpose is to create a forceful burst of air that may dislodge the object.

4. Check after each blow to see if the object has been dislodged. If not, continue giving up to five back blows.

The key here is force—don't be afraid to hit hard enough to create the necessary pressure to clear the airway. However, you should be careful not to use so much force that it causes injury, especially with smaller individuals like children or infants.

When to Use Abdominal Thrusts

If back blows do not clear the obstruction, the next step is abdominal thrusts. This technique involves applying pressure just below the person's ribcage to force the object out. Here's how you can perform abdominal thrusts:

1. Stand behind the choking individual.

2. Place your arms around their waist and make a fist with one hand.

3. Position your fist just above the navel, with the thumb side against their abdomen.

4. Grasp your fist with your other hand and pull sharply inward and upward. The motion should be quick and forceful, as if trying to lift them slightly off the ground.

5. Perform up to five abdominal thrusts, checking between each one to see if the obstruction has been removed.

Abdominal thrusts are particularly effective when the object is lodged deeper in the airway and back blows are not successful. However, it's crucial to use the correct amount of force to avoid injuring the person, especially in smaller adults and children. For infants under a year old, abdominal thrusts should be avoided, as their organs are more vulnerable. Instead, you should perform chest thrusts using two fingers in the center of the chest, just below the nipple line.

When to Alternate Between Techniques

If you've given five back blows and the object hasn't cleared, move on to five abdominal thrusts. Alternating between back blows and abdominal thrusts can help dislodge the object by applying different types of pressure on the airway. Continue this cycle until the object is cleared, or until the person becomes unconscious.

It's also important to understand that these techniques can be physically tiring, so if possible, ask someone else nearby to assist while you continue your efforts. Call emergency services as soon as possible if the object is not dislodged quickly, especially if the person becomes unresponsive.

Handling an Unconscious Person

If the person becomes unconscious due to choking, lay them flat on the ground and begin chest compressions, similar to CPR. Chest compressions can sometimes help dislodge an object, so check the mouth for the object before each breath. If you see it, carefully remove it without pushing it further down the throat.

Performing Back Blows and Thrusts on Different Age Groups

For adults and children over one year, the combination of back blows and abdominal thrusts is the standard approach. However, for infants under one year, you should adjust your technique. For choking infants, use five gentle back blows, followed by five chest thrusts, repeating the cycle until the object is cleared or help arrives.

Make sure to support the baby's head, and never use excessive force on their fragile bodies. Lay the baby face down along your arm and give firm but gentle back blows. Flip them over to perform chest thrusts by pressing with two fingers in the middle of the chest. The techniques are similar, but the force and precision need to be adjusted based on the size and fragility of the infant.

Aftercare for the Person

Even if the object is successfully removed, the person may still have some lingering symptoms. They could have a sore throat, trouble swallowing, or feel shaken by the experience. It's always a good idea to seek medical advice after a choking incident, especially if abdominal thrusts were performed, as these can sometimes cause internal injuries.

Extra Tips

Always stay calm in a choking situation, as panic can make things worse. Keep in mind that prevention is key—small objects, nuts, and hard candies can be choking hazards, especially for children. Educate those around you on the importance of chewing food thoroughly and avoiding talking while eating to reduce the risk of choking. Finally, taking a first aid class can help you practice these life-saving techniques.

Chapter 8: First Aid for Shock

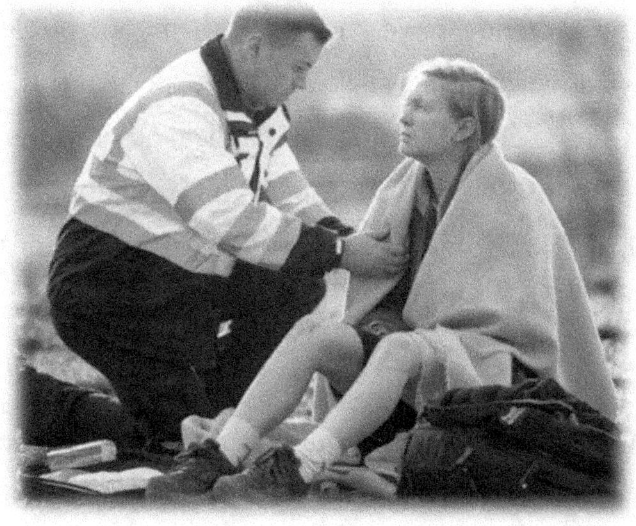

Tragedy befell the Johnson family when their 17-year-old son, Jack, was severely injured in a car accident. Despite apparent minor wounds, Jack rapidly deteriorated due to untreated shock. Unrecognized by bystanders, Jack's pale skin, rapid heartbeat, and shallow breathing signaled impending collapse. As precious minutes ticked by, Jack's condition worsened, leading to organ failure and eventual loss of life. This devastating outcome underscores the critical importance of recognizing and responding to shock. Simple first aid interventions could have potentially saved Jack's life.

Daily, Weekly, and Monthly Coop Cleaning Routines

Keeping your chicken coop clean is essential not only for the health of your flock but also for managing odors and preventing pests. By setting up a regular cleaning routine—daily, weekly, and monthly—you can ensure that your chickens live in a sanitary environment that minimizes the risk of disease. It might seem like a big task at first, but once you get into the rhythm of things, it becomes part of your routine. Here's a detailed guide on how to manage each type of cleaning and keep your coop in top shape.

Daily Cleaning Routine

The daily cleaning tasks are all about maintaining basic hygiene. These small steps prevent bigger issues down the line, like strong odors or a buildup of bacteria. One of the first things you should do each morning is to check the water supply. Make sure that the water is fresh and that the container is free of dirt or algae. Water can easily become contaminated with droppings, bedding, or feed, so it's important to dump out old water, rinse the container, and refill it with fresh water each day.

Along with water, inspect the feeders to ensure that they aren't clogged with wet or moldy feed. You don't need to refill the feeder every day if it's not empty, but it's a good idea to clean out any debris that may have fallen into the feed. Wet food can lead to mold growth, which poses a health hazard to your chickens.

Another essential part of daily cleaning is managing droppings. Chickens naturally produce a significant amount of waste, and while you can't avoid that, you can manage it effectively. Each day, remove visible droppings from areas like roosting bars or high-traffic areas in the coop. If your coop has a dropping board under the roosts, scrape it clean. This helps to cut down on odors and makes your weekly cleaning easier.

Weekly Cleaning Routine

Weekly cleaning is where you tackle deeper cleaning tasks to prevent the spread of bacteria and pests. Start by focusing on the bedding. Most chicken coops have bedding made of straw, wood shavings, or sand. While you don't need to change all the bedding every week, you should remove any particularly dirty or wet areas, especially around nesting boxes and under roosts. Fresh bedding should be added to maintain a clean environment for the chickens to nest and rest.

Next, pay attention to the coop's ventilation system. Over time, dust, feathers, and dirt can build up, clogging any air vents. This can lead to poor air circulation, which isn't healthy for your chickens, especially in hotter climates. Clean the vents and any windows to ensure that fresh air flows freely through the coop.

Take time each week to scrub and clean the waterers and feeders with warm, soapy water. This helps remove bacteria and prevents any buildup of grime. Let the containers air dry thoroughly before refilling them to avoid creating a moist environment where mold or mildew could develop. In addition to scrubbing, inspect the coop for any signs of damage, like loose nails, splintered wood, or holes. It's better to fix these minor issues early rather than allow them to turn into bigger problems.

Monthly Cleaning Routine

Your monthly coop cleaning is when you perform a deep clean to reset the coop and make sure it's a healthy space for your chickens to thrive. Begin by removing all of the bedding from the coop, including what's in the nesting boxes and under the roosts. This is important because bedding can trap moisture and harbor bacteria over time. Once the old bedding is out, sweep the floors thoroughly to remove any remaining debris.

After sweeping, it's time to disinfect the coop. Use a safe cleaning solution, such as a mixture of vinegar and water, to scrub the floors, walls, and nesting boxes. Be sure to get into any corners or small crevices where droppings or dirt may have accumulated. While scrubbing, keep an eye out for any signs of pests like mites or lice, as a thorough monthly cleaning is your best chance to catch these problems before they affect your flock. Once everything is scrubbed down, allow the coop to dry completely before adding new bedding.

Monthly cleaning is also the perfect time to inspect your coop's structural integrity. Check for signs of wear and tear, especially in areas that get a lot of traffic, such as door hinges, locks, or perches. Ensure that everything is secure, as gaps or holes in the structure could invite predators or pests into the coop. Also, double-check your nesting boxes to see if they need any repairs or fresh bedding.

Lastly, deep clean and sanitize the feeders and waterers during your monthly routine. While you should be cleaning them weekly, giving them a thorough scrub and disinfecting them monthly ensures that they remain free of harmful bacteria. Properly maintaining these items helps to prevent diseases that could otherwise spread quickly through the flock.

Extra Tips

To keep your coop in the best shape, consider using a method called the deep litter system, where you allow bedding to decompose slightly, forming a compost layer that keeps your coop warm in colder months. It also reduces how often you need to do a full clean. Just remember to regularly add fresh bedding to the top. If you follow these routines diligently, your coop will remain clean, safe, and comfortable for your chickens.

Managing Odors and Pests in the Coop

Keeping your chicken coop clean and odor-free is not just about comfort—it's essential for the health of your chickens. Unpleasant smells can attract pests like flies, rodents, and other predators, making the environment unsanitary. Taking proactive steps to control odors and keep pests at bay is critical for maintaining a healthy coop. Managing these factors requires a balance between regular cleaning, proper ventilation, and pest control techniques. By focusing on these areas, you can create a clean, safe, and odor-free space for your flock.

First, controlling odors begins with addressing the root cause: chicken waste. Droppings are high in ammonia, and when left to accumulate, they release strong odors that can lead to respiratory issues for your chickens. A regular cleaning schedule is the key to minimizing this problem. Daily cleaning, such as scraping droppings off perches and collecting any waste around the coop, can help significantly. However, weekly deep cleaning is essential to really tackle odors. This involves changing the bedding, cleaning nesting boxes, and disinfecting surfaces where droppings might accumulate.

Choosing the right bedding material also plays a huge role in controlling odors. Straw, pine shavings, and wood chips are popular options, but each has its advantages. Pine shavings are particularly absorbent and can help reduce moisture, which is a major contributor to bad smells. When you select a bedding material, consider how well it absorbs both droppings and moisture. The more absorbent the bedding, the better it will be at reducing odors in your coop.

Ventilation is another critical factor in keeping the coop fresh. Good airflow helps carry away ammonia fumes and other unpleasant smells, keeping the environment breathable for your chickens. Ensure that your coop has sufficient windows or vents that allow air to circulate, even in colder months. If your coop doesn't have enough ventilation, you may notice a build-up of smells no matter how clean you keep it. During the summer, larger openings can be helpful, while in the winter, adjustable vents can let fresh air in without letting too much cold in.

Next, you'll need to address the issue of pests. Chickens naturally attract pests like flies, mites, and rodents, especially when there is food and waste present. To minimize pests, focus on reducing their access to both. Store feed in sealed containers to prevent attracting rodents. Any spillage should be cleaned up immediately, and food bowls should be removed from the coop at night to avoid inviting unwanted visitors. Rodents are drawn to easy food sources, so keeping the feeding area clean is crucial.

Flies are another common problem in coops, particularly in the warmer months. They are attracted to chicken droppings and can quickly become overwhelming if not controlled. Using fly traps around the coop can be an effective way to keep their numbers down. Additionally, some natural deterrents, like hanging herbs such as mint or lavender, can help keep flies away. Installing screens over ventilation areas can also reduce the chances of flies entering the coop, and applying diatomaceous earth to areas prone to fly activity can make the environment less attractive to them.

Mites and lice can also pose a threat to your chickens' health. These pests can cause skin irritation and lead to feather loss or even illness if left untreated. A common way to prevent mites and lice is to provide your chickens with access to a dust bath. Dust bathing is a natural behavior for chickens, and it helps them keep their feathers clean while discouraging mites from settling in. You can encourage this by offering a dusting area filled with dirt, sand, or diatomaceous earth. Regularly check your chickens for signs of mites, such as excessive scratching or bald spots.

Cleaning and disinfecting your coop regularly will also help keep pests at bay. Pay particular attention to nesting boxes, as these areas can be hotspots for mites and other pests. Replace the bedding in these areas often and use a natural or poultry-safe disinfectant to clean surfaces. For extra pest control, you can sprinkle diatomaceous earth in the bedding and nesting areas, as this can kill off mites and other small pests without harming your chickens.

Finally, keeping your coop dry is essential for managing both odors and pests. Damp bedding is a breeding ground for bacteria and attracts pests like flies and rodents. If the coop gets wet during rainy seasons or because of spilled water, it's important to address the moisture right away. Placing the coop in a well-drained area and using tarps or other coverings to protect it from rain can help keep it dry. Make sure the waterers in the coop are not leaking, and if they are, replace them with better-sealed models.

Extra Tip:

Consider using natural odor-neutralizing products, such as barn lime or zeolite, which can be sprinkled over bedding to absorb moisture and reduce ammonia smells. These products are safe for chickens and can greatly help in keeping odors under control.

Tips for winter and Summer Coop Maintenance

Maintaining a chicken coop throughout the changing seasons is vital for keeping your flock safe, healthy, and comfortable. Each season brings its own set of challenges, but with proper care, you can create an environment that supports your chickens' well-being. This section provides practical tips for maintaining your coop during winter and summer, ensuring that your chickens thrive all year round.

Winter Coop Maintenance

As temperatures drop, your coop needs specific adjustments to keep your chickens warm and safe from harsh weather. Here are key steps to consider:

Insulation: Start by insulating the coop to help retain heat. Use materials like straw bales, foam boards, or reflective insulation. Make sure to insulate the walls, roof, and even the floor if possible. Ensure that ventilation is still maintained to prevent moisture build-up, which can lead to respiratory issues.

Bedding: A thick layer of bedding is crucial in winter. Use straw, wood shavings, or hemp to provide insulation from the cold ground. Regularly change the bedding to maintain cleanliness and reduce odors. The added bedding also helps in maintaining warmth as chickens scratch and move around.

Water Supply: Chickens need access to fresh water, even in winter. Use heated waterers or insulated containers to prevent freezing. Check the water supply frequently to ensure it's available and unfrozen. Hydration is essential for your chickens' health, especially in colder months.

Heat Sources: While chickens are generally hardy, providing a heat source can be beneficial in extreme cold. Consider using a safe heat lamp or ceramic heater designed for animal use. Place it in a corner of the coop, ensuring it's securely mounted and away from flammable materials.

Draft Protection: Ensure the coop is draft-free while still allowing for ventilation. Check for gaps or cracks in the walls and roof, and seal them with caulk or weather stripping. Use heavy curtains or tarps to block drafts on especially cold nights.

Monitoring Health: Keep an eye on your chickens during winter months. Watch for signs of frostbite on combs and wattles, which can occur in very low temperatures. If you notice any issues, separate the affected chickens and provide extra warmth and care.

Summer Coop Maintenance

As the temperatures rise, your coop will need adjustments to keep your chickens cool and comfortable. Here's how to prepare for summer heat:

Ventilation: Proper airflow is essential during hot weather. Install windows or vents that can be opened to increase air circulation. You may also want to use fans to help keep the air moving

inside the coop. Ensure the fans are chicken-
safe and do not pose a risk of injury.

Shade: Create shaded areas around the coop using tarps, trees, or umbrellas. This will help prevent overheating. Chickens will often seek shade during the hottest parts of the day, so providing these areas can help them stay cool and reduce heat stress.

Water Access: Just as in winter, hydration is critical during summer. Ensure that your chickens have access to fresh, cool water at all times. Consider placing multiple water sources in the coop and run to encourage them to drink more. You might also add ice to their water during particularly hot days.

Dust Bathing Areas: Chickens love to take dust baths, which helps keep their feathers clean and free from pests. Create designated dust bathing areas with loose, dry soil or sand. This will keep them comfortable and help regulate their body temperature.

Pest Control: Warm weather can bring more pests like flies and mites. Regularly clean the coop and surrounding areas to prevent infestations. Use natural repellents like diatomaceous earth in nesting boxes and dusting areas to help control pests without harmful chemicals.

Health Checks: During the summer, monitor your chickens for signs of heat stress, such as excessive panting, lethargy, or drooping wings. If you notice any symptoms, move them to a cooler area, provide fresh water, and consider adding electrolyte solutions to help them recover.

General Maintenance Tips

Regardless of the season, there are general maintenance practices you should follow to ensure your coop remains in good condition:

Regular Cleaning: Keeping your coop clean is essential for the health of your chickens. Remove droppings and old bedding regularly. A clean coop helps prevent the spread of diseases and keeps odors in check.

Inspection: Frequently check the coop for any damage, such as broken boards or loose wire. Repairing these issues promptly can prevent accidents and provide a safer environment for your flock.

Proper Feeding: Ensure your chickens receive a balanced diet throughout the year. Adjust their feed according to the season, as their nutritional needs may change with the weather.

By taking these steps to maintain your chicken coop during both winter and summer, you create a healthier and safer environment for your flock. Regular upkeep not only ensures their comfort but also contributes to their overall productivity and happiness.

Extra Tips

-Invest in a good quality thermometer to monitor the temperature inside the coop. This can help you make timely adjustments.

-During the summer, consider providing frozen treats made from fruits or vegetables mixed with water to keep your chickens cool and entertained.

-Keep a first aid kit handy for any minor injuries or health issues that may arise due to seasonal changes.

-Educate yourself about the specific breeds of chickens you have, as some may have unique needs regarding temperature and care.

Taking the time to care for your coop in different seasons can make a significant difference in your chickens' health and productivity. Your efforts will result in a thriving flock that can enjoy all the benefits of a well-maintained environment.

Chapter 9: Dealing with Poisoning

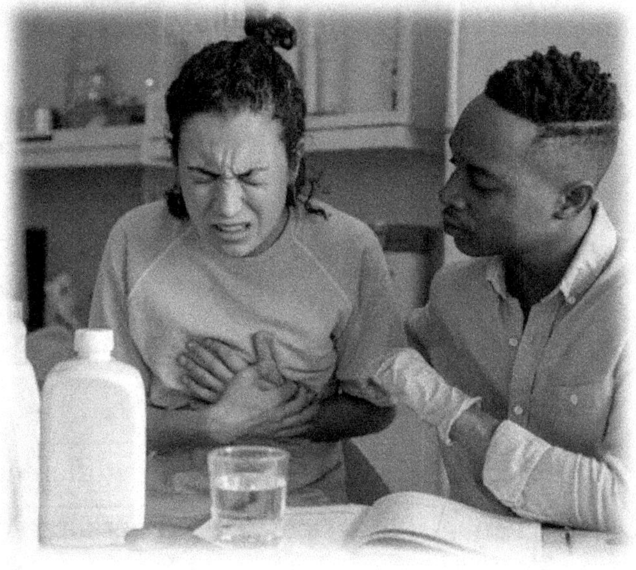

Tragedy struck when two-year-old Olivia ingested her grandmother's medication. Panicked, her grandmother gave Olivia a glass of milk, hoping to neutralize the poison. Unbeknownst to her, this worsened the situation. Delaying medical attention, Olivia's condition rapidly deteriorated. By the time she reached the hospital, irreversible damage had occurred, leaving Olivia with permanent neurological damage. This heartbreaking incident highlights the dangers of improper poisoning response. Knowing the correct procedures – calling the poison control hotline and seeking immediate medical attention – could have prevented this devastating outcome.

Identifying the Source of Poisoning

When faced with a situation involving potential poisoning, your immediate actions can be crucial. Knowing how to identify the source of poisoning not only aids in determining the appropriate first aid response but also helps medical professionals provide the best treatment. This section will guide you through the signs to look for and steps to take in order to effectively identify the source of poisoning.

Identifying poisoning starts with a thorough assessment of the situation. You should observe the person affected and gather as much information as possible. Pay attention to their symptoms, the environment, and any substances that may have been involved. Common signs of poisoning can include nausea, vomiting, difficulty breathing, altered consciousness, and skin irritations. These symptoms may vary depending on the type of poison and the amount that was ingested, inhaled, or absorbed.

First, you need to determine what the person has been exposed to. Look around the area for any unusual substances or containers. This can include household cleaners, medications, chemicals, or plants. If you suspect poisoning from a particular substance, check for labels or packaging that can provide vital information. Many products will have warning labels or safety data that can indicate whether they are toxic.

If the person was outside, consider potential environmental poisons. Pesticides, herbicides, and certain plants can be harmful if ingested or even touched. Familiarize yourself with common poisonous plants in your area, such as oleander, foxglove, or deadly nightshade. Knowing these can help you quickly identify a potential threat.

In cases of suspected drug overdose, gather information about any medications the person has taken. This includes prescription drugs, over-the-counter medications, or illegal substances. If possible, have the medication containers available for medical responders to assess. Look for empty bottles, pill packs, or any drug paraphernalia. Even small quantities of certain substances can cause serious harm, so your ability to identify what has been ingested can be lifesaving.

For inhalation poisoning, try to determine the source of the fumes. This may include smoke from a fire, carbon monoxide from a faulty heater, or chemicals from cleaning products. If the person is unconscious or unable to communicate, ask anyone nearby if they noticed any unusual smells or substances before the incident occurred. If you're in a confined space and suspect carbon monoxide exposure, evacuate the area immediately while ensuring your own safety.

When assessing poisoning, keep in mind the time of exposure. Timing can be crucial for determining the right treatment. If you know when the substance was ingested, inhaled, or absorbed, communicate this information to medical professionals. They can provide the necessary care more effectively if they know how much time has passed since the exposure occurred.

Next, it's essential to gather information about the affected person's medical history. This includes any known allergies, existing medical conditions, or ongoing medications. This information is valuable for medical responders and can guide them in determining the best course of action. If the person is unconscious or unable to provide this information, ask family members or friends who may know.

Once you have gathered all this information, contact emergency services or a poison control center immediately. While you wait for help to arrive, continue monitoring the person's condition. If they become unresponsive or show signs of distress, be prepared to provide first aid measures such as CPR, if necessary.

It's vital to avoid inducing vomiting unless specifically instructed by a medical professional or poison control. Some substances can cause more damage if they are brought back up. Instead, focus on providing accurate information to those who can help.

To help you in such situations, here are some extra tips: Always keep your home stocked with emergency contact numbers for local poison control and emergency services. Familiarize yourself with the common poisons in your household and read labels carefully. Keeping a first aid kit that includes activated charcoal can also be beneficial, but use it only under the guidance of a medical professional. Remember, your awareness and quick action can make all the difference in a poisoning emergency.

First Aid for Ingested, Inhaled, and Absorbed Poisons

When it comes to emergencies involving poison, knowing how to act quickly and effectively can make a significant difference. Poisoning can occur through various means, including ingestion, inhalation, and absorption. Each method requires a different approach in terms of first aid, but understanding the signs and steps to take can help you manage the situation calmly and effectively. In this section, you'll learn about the different types of poisoning, how to recognize symptoms, and the appropriate first aid measures to take.

Recognizing poisoning symptoms is the first step in addressing the issue. The signs can vary depending on the type of poison and how it entered the body. Common symptoms include nausea, vomiting, abdominal pain, confusion, difficulty breathing, or skin reactions. If someone has ingested a poison, you may notice changes in their behavior, like irritability or lethargy. If the poison was inhaled, they may show signs of respiratory distress, such as coughing, wheezing, or difficulty breathing. For absorbed poisons, look for redness, swelling, or a rash on the skin.

Ingested Poisons:

If someone has swallowed a poison, the first thing you should do is stay calm. Try to gather as much information as possible, such as what the person ingested, how much they consumed, and when it happened. This information is crucial for medical professionals. Do not induce vomiting unless instructed to do so by a poison control center or a medical professional. Inducing vomiting can sometimes because more harm, especially if the poison is caustic (like bleach or drain cleaner) or if the person is unconscious or having difficulty breathing.

If the person is conscious and alert, you may give them a small amount of water or milk to drink. This can help dilute the poison and minimize its effects. However, avoid giving anything acidic, such as fruit juice, as it can worsen the situation. If the person is unconscious or having seizures, do not attempt to give them anything by mouth.

Once you've stabilized the individual, it's essential to seek professional help. Contact your local emergency services or a poison control center immediately. Provide them with all the information you gathered, as this will assist them in determining the best course of action.

Inhaled Poisons:

Inhalation of toxic substances can occur in various situations, such as exposure to fumes from chemicals, smoke, or carbon monoxide. If someone has inhaled a poison, the priority is to get them to fresh air immediately. Move the person away from the source of the poison while ensuring your safety.

Once in fresh air, check for breathing. If the person is struggling to breathe or showing signs of distress, it's crucial to call emergency services right away. In the meantime, help the individual sit in a comfortable position, ideally with their knees bent to alleviate any pressure on the abdomen. Encourage them to take slow, deep breaths if they can.

If the person loses consciousness or stops breathing, be prepared to perform CPR. If trained, administer CPR until emergency personnel arrive or until the person regains consciousness. If you have access to an automated external defibrillator (AED), use it if needed.

Absorbed Poisons:

Absorption poisoning occurs when a toxic substance comes into contact with the skin. This can happen through pesticides, certain plants, or chemicals. If you suspect someone has absorbed a poison, the first step is to remove the contaminated clothing and rinse the affected area with running water for at least 15-20 minutes. This helps to wash away the poison from the skin and reduces the risk of further absorption.

While rinsing, be careful not to scrub the area, as this can cause the poison to penetrate deeper into the skin. If the individual is experiencing a severe reaction, such as difficulty breathing or swelling, call for emergency assistance immediately.

For eye exposure, if a toxic substance gets into someone's eyes, you need to flush the eyes gently with clean, running water for at least 15 minutes. Ensure the person is looking in the opposite direction of the water flow to avoid washing the poison into the unaffected eye. After rinsing, seek medical attention.

Extra Tips for Handling Poisoning Emergencies

In emergencies involving poison, preparation and knowledge are key. Here are some additional tips to keep in mind:

Know Your Poisons: Familiarize yourself with common household poisons, including cleaning agents, medications, and plants. Keeping a list of these items can be helpful in emergencies.

Keep Emergency Numbers Handy: Have the contact information for your local poison control center and emergency services easily accessible.

Stay Calm: Your calm demeanor can help reassure the affected person and ensure that you can think clearly during a crisis.

Act Quickly: Time is of the essence in poison-related emergencies. Acting swiftly can help minimize the effects of the poison.

By being informed and prepared, you can play a critical role in addressing poisoning incidents effectively and ensuring that the affected person receives the necessary help.

Managing Poisoning in Children

When it comes to children's safety, understanding how to manage poisoning is vital. Children are naturally curious and often explore their surroundings without fully grasping the dangers. They may accidentally ingest household products, medications, or other harmful substances. Recognizing the signs of poisoning, knowing how to respond effectively, and taking preventive measures can save lives and minimize harm. This section will provide you with practical guidelines on how to handle situations involving poisoning in children.

To begin, it's crucial to recognize the signs of poisoning in children. Symptoms can vary widely depending on the substance ingested, but there are common indicators to watch for. Look for unusual behavior such as excessive drooling, difficulty breathing, or drowsiness. Other symptoms may include vomiting, abdominal pain, or changes in skin color. If you notice these signs, it is essential to act quickly.

The first step in managing poisoning is to assess the situation. Remain calm and try to determine what your child has ingested. Check for any labels on the product or packaging and take note of the name and active ingredients. If possible, bring this information with you when seeking medical help. Avoid inducing vomiting unless specifically directed to do so by a healthcare professional. In some cases, inducing vomiting can cause more harm than good.

If your child is conscious and alert, ask them what they consumed and how much. This information will be vital for medical professionals in determining the appropriate treatment. If they are unconscious or having seizures, call emergency services immediately. While waiting for help, ensure your child is in a safe position. Place them on their side to prevent choking, and monitor their breathing and responsiveness.

In many cases, prompt medical intervention is crucial. If you suspect poisoning, contact your local poison control center or seek immediate medical attention. Keep the phone number for your local poison control center handy for quick access. When you call, provide them with all the information you have gathered, including your child's age, weight, the substance involved, and any symptoms observed.

If the poisoning involves a chemical or household product, do not attempt to treat your child at home. Many substances can react negatively when treated improperly. For example, some cleaners may cause more damage if vomited. Medical professionals have access to specific antidotes and treatments tailored for different types of poison, so it is vital to get your child to a medical facility as quickly as possible.

Prevention is the best strategy when it comes to poisoning in children. Take proactive measures to reduce the risk of poisoning in your home.

Start by storing all medications, cleaning supplies, and chemicals out of reach or in locked cabinets. Always keep these items in their original containers with clear labels, and never transfer them to food or drink containers, as this can lead to accidental ingestion.

Educate your child about the dangers of certain substances, even at a young age. Teach them to ask an adult before tasting or touching unfamiliar items. Use age-appropriate language and examples to help them understand the potential risks. As they grow older, reinforce these lessons by discussing the importance of safety and the harmful effects of ingesting unknown substances.

It's also beneficial to regularly review your home for potential hazards. Conduct a thorough check of areas where hazardous materials are stored. Ensure that items like batteries, alcohol, and medications are secured. Consider using safety locks for cabinets and drawers to add an extra layer of protection.

In case of a poisoning incident, keep essential items on hand to facilitate a quick response. Have the contact numbers for your local poison control center and nearby medical facilities readily accessible. Create a first aid kit that includes necessary items such as activated charcoal (only for use under medical guidance), gloves, and a thermometer. Having these supplies prepared can help you respond more effectively in an emergency.

Lastly, it is important to stay calm during a poisoning incident. Your reaction can significantly impact how your child responds to the situation. By staying composed, you can think clearly and act swiftly. Children often take cues from adults, and your ability to manage the situation calmly can help reassure them.

Extra Tips:

- Always keep the poison control center number easily accessible.

- Consider taking a first aid and CPR course to be better prepared for emergencies.

- Regularly review and practice emergency plans with your family.

- Encourage open discussions about safety and potential dangers with your children. This can help reinforce their understanding and promote a culture of safety at home.

Chapter 10: First Aid for Breathing Emergencies

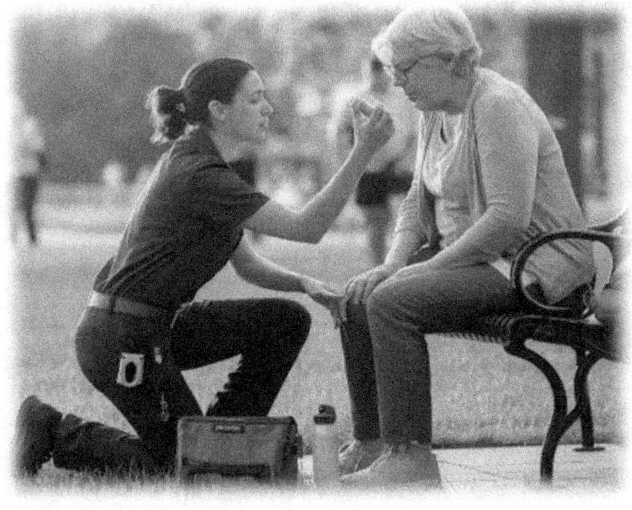

Tragedy befell the Jason family when their 45-year-old father, Armstrong suffered an asthma attack at a family gathering. Unfamiliar with breathing emergency protocols, his relatives mistakenly administered oxygen incorrectly and delayed calling 911. As Armstrong's condition worsened, they attempted to give him medication that was past its expiration date. The lack of proper intervention led to respiratory failure, resulting in Armstrong's untimely death. This devastating outcome underscores the critical importance of recognizing breathing emergencies and responding with evidence-based first aid techniques.

Checking Local Laws and Regulations for Backyard Chickens

Before raising backyard chickens, it's essential to understand the local laws and regulations that govern poultry keeping in your area. These rules exist to ensure public safety, animal welfare, and neighborhood harmony. Checking and adhering to these laws is a crucial first step in becoming a responsible chicken owner, saving you potential legal trouble down the road.

To start, you'll need to investigate the specific rules in your city or town. Local ordinances, zoning regulations, and even homeowners' association (HOA) rules can impact what is allowed. Each area has its unique requirements, so thorough research is key. Begin by contacting your local municipality or visiting their website, where many provide zoning laws and guidelines related to keeping chickens. Some cities may permit backyard chickens with little restriction, while others may have strict limitations on the number of birds you can keep, where you can house them, and how you maintain their environment.

In many urban or suburban areas, local zoning codes dictate whether you're allowed to keep chickens at all. Zoning laws typically classify properties by how they can be used: residential, agricultural, or commercial. Chickens, as livestock, often fall under agricultural zoning, but some municipalities have made exceptions, allowing residents in suburban or even urban zones to keep a small flock of hens. For example, you may live in a residential zone where chickens are allowed, but roosters—due to noise complaints—are not.

A good place to begin your search is the local government or city hall, where zoning maps and legal codes are available. Municipal websites are another great resource, as they often publish updated information regarding backyard chickens. If the regulations are unclear, reaching out to the zoning or planning office in person or via phone can provide clarity. Make sure you're specific when asking about keeping backyard chickens, as laws about other pets or agricultural animals might not apply to chickens.

Once you've confirmed that your zoning laws allow chickens, check for restrictions on the number of birds. Some areas may allow only three or four chickens per household, while others might permit more depending on property size. Cities may also regulate how far your chicken coop must be from neighboring properties or buildings. These rules are in place to prevent nuisances such as odor, noise, and pests from disturbing the community. Be prepared to comply with these guidelines, as they may require you to rethink your coop's location. A setback rule might state that your coop needs to be at least 10 feet away from any neighboring property line.

Noise ordinances are another common regulation, particularly regarding roosters. Many urban areas have banned roosters altogether, as their crowing can be disruptive. If you're keen on getting chickens primarily for eggs, you won't need roosters, since hens can lay eggs without them. However, if you do want to keep a rooster for breeding purposes, double-check that local ordinances permit it.

Additionally, there may be regulations concerning the type of enclosure you use for your chickens. Most places require chicken coops to be built to certain standards to prevent the spread of disease, protect the chickens from predators, and minimize odors. The coop should be secure, well-ventilated, and easy to clean. You might also need to get a permit to build a coop, especially if it exceeds a specific size. When in doubt, consult your city's building department for advice on what's acceptable and required. If your neighborhood is part of an HOA, be sure to check with them as well, since they often have their own set of rules that may be even more restrictive than city laws.

Another crucial aspect is the health and safety regulations governing poultry. Many areas require backyard chicken owners to register their flock with the local agricultural department. This registration helps monitor potential disease outbreaks, such as avian flu, which can spread rapidly among birds. Local laws may also require that you keep your chickens vaccinated against certain diseases. Keeping up with these health regulations ensures the safety of your chickens and helps prevent issues that could affect your neighborhood or even the wider poultry population.

It's also worth investigating waste management rules. Some municipalities have specific guidelines on how to dispose of chicken waste, which can be used as compost but must be handled properly to avoid attracting pests or causing environmental harm. Maintaining a clean coop is not only good for the health of your chickens but also helps you comply with local waste regulations.

Beyond city or municipal laws, you should also consider state laws and animal welfare regulations. Many states have laws prohibiting animal cruelty, which apply to how you care for your chickens. These regulations ensure that chickens are provided with adequate food, water, and shelter, and that they are treated humanely. It's important to familiarize yourself with these requirements as well to avoid any legal pitfalls.

Lastly, you might encounter community concerns when keeping backyard chickens, especially if you live in a densely populated area. It's a good idea to communicate with your neighbors before starting your backyard chicken venture. Letting them know your plans and assuring them that you'll be responsible with noise and cleanliness can go a long way in maintaining good relationships and preventing complaints.

Extra Tips

To make your experience easier, consider keeping records of all permits and registrations related to your chickens. This will help you stay organized and avoid potential penalties. Always remember that raising chickens responsibly not only benefits you but also contributes to a cleaner, healthier community.

Keeping the Peace with Neighbors: Noise and Odor Control

Living in close quarters with neighbors can be a rewarding experience, but it also comes with responsibilities, especially when raising chickens. If you keep chickens in your backyard, managing noise and odor becomes critical to maintaining a peaceful relationship with your neighbors. While chickens are generally low-maintenance, their presence can still cause disruptions if the noise or smell from your coop is not properly managed. This section will cover practical tips for keeping your chickens from becoming a nuisance to your neighbors.

Managing Noise from Chickens

Chickens, particularly roosters, can be noisy, especially at dawn. While some noise is natural, excessive clucking, crowing, and squawking may disturb your neighbors, leading to complaints. To keep the peace, consider the following steps.

First, evaluate the size and breed of your flock. Roosters are typically the loudest members of a chicken coop, known for crowing at all hours. If possible, avoid keeping roosters unless necessary for breeding purposes. Many municipalities have restrictions on keeping roosters within city limits due to noise concerns. If you already own a rooster, you can try using a "no-crow" collar, which is designed to reduce the volume of a rooster's crow without harming the bird.

Beyond roosters, hens can also be vocal, especially when laying eggs or if they feel threatened. However, hens are generally quieter than roosters, so managing their environment can help reduce unnecessary noise. Ensure they feel safe in their coop, with adequate space and proper nesting boxes, as overcrowding or discomfort can lead to increased vocalizations. Additionally, placing the coop as far from your neighbors' property as possible can help minimize the impact of any noise.

Creating a routine for your chickens can also reduce early morning noise. Chickens tend to be most vocal when the sun rises. By using blackout curtains in their coop, you can delay their exposure to daylight, encouraging them to stay quieter longer in the morning. Feeding them shortly after they wake up can also distract them and keep them content, further reducing noise.

Lastly, consider soundproofing the coop. Adding insulation to the walls and roof can help muffle the sounds your chickens make, keeping the noise from traveling to neighboring homes. You should also perform regular checks to ensure there are no gaps or openings in the coop that allow sound to escape more easily.

Controlling Odor in the Coop

Another common concern when keeping chickens is the smell. Chicken waste can create a strong odor if the coop is not cleaned regularly, which can upset neighbors and make your yard an unpleasant place to be. Proper waste management and cleaning routines are crucial in keeping the odor at bay.

First, make sure you have an effective bedding material in the coop. Straw, wood shavings, and sand are all good options that help absorb moisture and minimize the smell. The deep litter method, where you allow bedding to compost inside the coop while periodically adding fresh layers, can also help manage odor while cutting down on cleaning frequency. The composting process helps break down chicken manure naturally, reducing the smell and providing nutrient-rich material for gardening when properly managed.

Another way to reduce odor is to ensure your coop has good ventilation. Poor air circulation can trap smells inside the coop, making the odor more noticeable. By installing vents at the top of the coop, you allow fresh air to enter while allowing ammonia and other odors to escape. This simple addition can make a significant difference in air quality, both inside and outside the coop.

Regular cleaning is essential to prevent buildup of waste and odor. Remove droppings and soiled bedding at least once a week, and replace the bedding to keep the coop fresh. If you're using the deep litter method, turn the bedding regularly to promote composting and prevent it from becoming compacted. Additionally, use odor-neutralizing products, like agricultural lime or coop-specific deodorizers, to control the smell. These can be sprinkled over bedding or placed in strategic areas to keep unpleasant odors at bay.

Cleaning the chicken run is just as important. Waste and food scraps left outside can lead to a strong smell and attract pests. Regularly rake the run and remove any waste or old food. If possible, create a separate compost pile for chicken manure that is far from your neighbors' property to prevent the smell from reaching their homes.

Considerate Placement and Communication

An often overlooked factor in keeping the peace with your neighbors is the placement of your coop. Before building or relocating your coop, try to place it as far from property lines as possible. This ensures that noise and odor are less likely to reach your neighbors. Fencing and tall hedges can also serve as barriers, helping to block noise and smells from traveling too far.

In addition to practical steps, open communication with your neighbors can go a long way. Let them know ahead of time that you plan to keep chickens, and listen to their concerns. By being proactive, you can address potential issues before they become problems. It's also a good idea to periodically check in with your neighbors to ensure that the noise or odor isn't bothering them.

Extra Tips

To keep the peace, always stay one step ahead of potential problems. For instance, keep a cleaning schedule and stick to it, so the coop doesn't become overwhelming. Try using herbs like lavender or mint around the coop to keep it smelling fresh, as they are known for their odor-reducing properties. These small touches can make a big difference in how your chickens are perceived in the neighborhood, ensuring that everyone enjoys a peaceful environment.

How to Administer Inhalers and Other Respiratory Aids

Understanding how to properly administer inhalers and other respiratory aids is an essential part of first aid, especially for individuals dealing with asthma or respiratory distress. These tools can make a huge difference in a medical emergency and offer immediate relief when used correctly. Knowing the right steps ensures that you can provide timely care and help prevent complications.

Administering inhalers is common in cases of asthma or when someone experiences shortness of breath due to other respiratory conditions. You might come across two types of inhalers: metered-dose inhalers (MDI), which deliver a specific amount of medicine in a puff, and dry powder inhalers (DPI), which release medication when the user inhales. The most important thing to remember when using an inhaler is ensuring that the person gets the correct dose and inhales the medication properly. To do this, you should first check the device to ensure it is not damaged and the medication is up to date.

Steps for Administering a Metered-Dose Inhaler (MDI):

1. **Preparation**: Before giving someone an inhaler, make sure they are sitting upright. This helps open the airway, making it easier for them to breathe. Shake the inhaler well, usually for about 5-10 seconds, to mix the medication inside.

2. **Attaching a Spacer (if available)**: A spacer is a helpful device, especially for people who struggle with inhalers. It attaches to the inhaler and holds the medication, allowing the user to take slow breaths. This ensures that the medicine reaches the lungs rather than getting stuck in the mouth or throat. If the person has a spacer, attach it to the inhaler before use.

3. **Inhalation**: If you're using an inhaler without a spacer, have the person place the mouthpiece into their mouth, sealing their lips

around it. Tell them to breathe out completely first, then, as they start to breathe in slowly, press the inhaler once to release the medication. They should continue breathing in for about 3-5 seconds to draw the medicine deeply into their lungs.

4. Holding the Breath: After inhaling the medication, instruct them to hold their breath for at least 10 seconds if possible. This allows the medicine to settle in their lungs and take effect. Afterward, they can exhale slowly.

5. Repeat if Necessary: Depending on the prescribed dose, you may need to give another puff. Wait about 30 seconds to 1 minute between doses if a second one is needed.

For dry powder inhalers (DPI), the process is slightly different. These inhalers don't require shaking, and instead of pressing down to release the medication, the person breathes in quickly and deeply through the mouthpiece. Remind them to keep their lips sealed around the mouthpiece and to take a deep, forceful breath to activate the medication. Again, holding the breath for around 10 seconds helps the medicine settle into the lungs.

What to Do After Administering an Inhaler:

Once the person has taken their medication, observe them closely to see if their breathing improves. Most people should feel relief within a few minutes, but if they don't, they may need additional treatment or medical attention. You can help them stay calm by encouraging slow, deep breaths. Anxiety can worsen breathing difficulties, so maintaining a calm atmosphere is essential.

Other Respiratory Aids:

In some cases, you might need to administer other types of respiratory aids, such as a nebulizer. A nebulizer turns liquid medication into a fine mist, making it easier to inhale. It's often used for people who are having severe asthma attacks or for children who can't use inhalers effectively. To use a nebulizer, attach the medication to the machine, and place the mask over the person's nose and mouth. Have them sit upright and breathe deeply as the nebulizer runs. This treatment usually takes about 5-10 minutes.

If someone is experiencing extreme respiratory distress and cannot breathe effectively on their own, you may need to administer oxygen if it's available. Oxygen should only be given if prescribed or under the guidance of emergency personnel. If you're in a situation where oxygen is needed, ensure the oxygen mask fits securely over the person's nose and mouth, adjusting the flow rate as instructed. Always monitor the person for improvement and be ready to call for emergency help if their condition does not improve.

Tips for Administering Respiratory Aids:

-**Stay Calm**: Staying calm during a respiratory emergency is crucial for both you and the person in distress. Encourage slow, deep breaths, which can also help reduce panic.

-Check the Device: Always ensure that the inhaler, spacer, or nebulizer is working correctly before use. If it's malfunctioning or expired, it won't deliver the necessary relief.

-Follow Up: After using an inhaler or nebulizer, check the person's condition every few minutes to ensure that the treatment is effective. If their condition worsens or they don't improve, seek medical assistance immediately.

Extra Tips

Knowing how to properly administer an inhaler or use a nebulizer can make a life-saving difference in respiratory emergencies. Always ensure the device is in good condition, and follow the steps carefully to deliver effective treatment. Extra tip: If you're helping someone who needs an inhaler regularly, suggest that they keep a spacer or second inhaler in convenient places like their bag or car for emergencies.

Chapter 11: Heat and Cold Emergencies

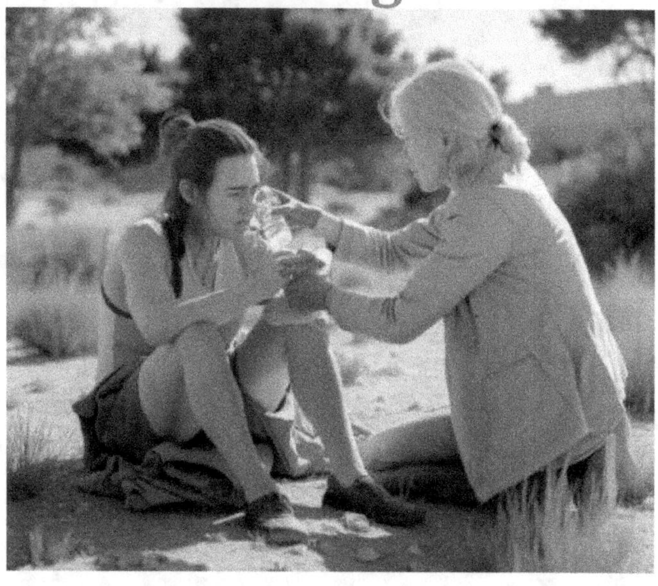

During a hiking trip, 19-year-old Alec ignored warnings about extreme heat and dehydration. When his friend, Lance, began showing symptoms of heatstroke – confusion, dizziness, and nausea – Alec gave him water to drink and encouraged him to keep hiking. Lance's condition rapidly worsened, leading to organ failure and permanent brain damage. The devastating outcome could have been prevented if Alex had recognized the signs of heat-related illness and provided proper care, such as cooling Lance's body and seeking immediate medical attention.

Treating Heat Exhaustion and Heatstroke

Heat-related emergencies can occur when your body is overwhelmed by high temperatures. Heat exhaustion and heatstroke are two common conditions that develop from prolonged exposure to heat, and both can be dangerous if not addressed promptly. Understanding how to treat these conditions is crucial, especially if you're in a hot climate or working outdoors. This section will guide you through identifying and managing heat exhaustion and heatstroke, helping you provide immediate care to someone in need.

Recognizing Heat Exhaustion

Heat exhaustion is your body's response to losing too much water and salt due to excessive sweating. This condition often develops after prolonged physical activity in hot, humid environments. The symptoms of heat exhaustion can vary but typically include heavy sweating, pale or clammy skin, muscle cramps, and a fast but weak pulse. You might also notice dizziness, nausea, or vomiting. It's important to act quickly when you notice these signs.

First, you'll want to move the person to a cooler area. Ideally, find a shaded spot or, if possible, an air-conditioned room. Make sure they rest and stop any strenuous activity to prevent their condition from worsening. Encourage them to drink cool water in small sips rather than large gulps. This helps the body rehydrate slowly and avoid further shock. If water is unavailable, an electrolyte drink can also be useful. Remove or loosen any tight clothing to allow better air circulation around the body.

Another effective way to cool the person down is to apply cool, wet cloths to their skin. Focus on areas like the neck, armpits, and forehead, as these spots tend to cool the body faster. You could also use a fan to help lower body temperature. If their symptoms persist for more than an hour or worsen, seek medical assistance immediately. While heat exhaustion is usually treatable at home, leaving it unchecked can lead to a more severe condition: heatstroke.

Identifying Heatstroke

Heatstroke is the more severe escalation of heat exhaustion, where the body's temperature rises to dangerous levels, typically above 104°F (40°C). This condition is a medical emergency and requires immediate intervention. The key difference between heat exhaustion and heatstroke is that in heatstroke, sweating often stops, and the person's skin may feel dry and hot to the touch. They may also become confused or disoriented, lose consciousness, or experience seizures. If left untreated, heatstroke can lead to organ damage or death.

The first step in treating heatstroke is calling emergency services immediately. While waiting for help, there are several things you can do to help stabilize the person's condition. Move them to a cooler area, as you would with heat exhaustion. However, in this case, you'll need to take more aggressive measures to cool their body. Remove excess clothing and begin actively cooling their body down with cold water. You can use a hose, a cool bath, or wet towels to bring their temperature down.

It's crucial to continuously monitor the person's body temperature if you have a thermometer. Aim to bring their temperature down to 102°F (39°C) or lower if possible. If they are conscious and able to drink, offer small sips of water. Be careful not to give them too much, as this can cause complications. If the person is unconscious or has a seizure, place them in the recovery position on their side. This helps to keep their airway open and reduces the risk of choking if they vomit.

Do not give aspirin or similar medications, as they can interfere with the body's heat regulation mechanisms. Remember that heatstroke can affect the brain and other vital organs, so even if the person seems to recover, medical professionals should evaluate them as soon as possible.

Preventing Heat-Related Illnesses

While treating heat exhaustion and heatstroke is essential, prevention is equally important. On particularly hot days, try to limit outdoor activities during the hottest parts of the day, usually between 10 a.m. and 4 p.m. If you must be outside, wear loose, light-colored clothing and a wide-brimmed hat to shield yourself from the sun. Hydration is also key—make sure to drink water regularly, even if you don't feel thirsty. If you're engaging in strenuous activity, take frequent breaks in a cool or shaded area.

Pay special attention to children, the elderly, and pets during hot weather, as they are more vulnerable to heat-related conditions. Never leave anyone in a parked car on a hot day, as temperatures can rise dangerously fast.

Long-Term Care after Heatstroke

After a person has suffered from heatstroke, they are more susceptible to heat-related illnesses in the future. Their recovery will require rest, hydration, and, in some cases, follow-up care to ensure there are no long-term complications. If the person has experienced organ damage or neurological symptoms, rehabilitation may be necessary.

Encourage them to avoid hot conditions as much as possible and to stay hydrated in the weeks following the incident. If they are planning to engage in any physical activity, it's important that they do so gradually, allowing their body time to adjust.

Extra Tips for Managing Heat-Related Emergencies

Preventing heat exhaustion and heatstroke starts with awareness. Keep an eye on weather reports during extreme heat and plan your activities accordingly. Wear sunscreen to protect your skin from sunburn, as damaged skin can impair the body's ability to cool down. If you're working outdoors, consider using a cooling vest or neck wrap to help regulate your body temperature. Finally, check on vulnerable individuals in your community during heatwaves to make sure they are staying cool and hydrated.

Heat emergencies can escalate quickly, but with the right preparation and immediate action, you can help prevent serious harm.

First Aid for Hypothermia and Frostbite

When temperatures drop significantly, the risk of hypothermia and frostbite increases. Understanding these conditions is essential for anyone who spends time outdoors in cold weather. This section will help you recognize the signs of hypothermia and frostbite, as well as guide you on how to provide first aid in these situations. Knowing how to respond quickly and effectively can save a life.

Hypothermia occurs when your body loses heat faster than it can produce it, causing your core temperature to drop dangerously low, typically below 95°F (35°C). This can happen even in relatively mild conditions, especially if you are wet or exposed to wind. Symptoms of hypothermia can vary, but they generally include intense shivering, confusion, drowsiness, weakness, and slurred speech. If left untreated, hypothermia can lead to serious complications, including heart failure and death.

Frostbite, on the other hand, is the freezing of body tissues, most commonly affecting the fingers, toes, ears, and nose. It occurs when the skin and underlying tissues freeze due to prolonged exposure to cold. The affected areas may appear red, white, or grayish-yellow and can feel numb. As frostbite progresses, the skin may become hard and blistered, and in severe cases, tissue can die, requiring medical intervention.

Recognizing Hypothermia

To effectively respond to hypothermia, you must first recognize its signs. Look for shivering, which is the body's initial response to cold. If the shivering stops, it could indicate a serious condition where the body is no longer able to generate heat. Confusion and disorientation are critical signs; the person may seem lethargic or unable to make decisions. They might also exhibit slurred speech, which can be alarming.

When assessing someone for hypothermia, check their skin temperature and color. The skin may feel cold to the touch and appear pale or blue. If the individual is conscious, ask how they feel. If they report feeling extremely cold, drowsy, or confused, you may need to act quickly.

Responding to Hypothermia

If you suspect someone is experiencing hypothermia, take immediate action. First, move the person to a warmer environment if possible. If indoors, remove any wet clothing and wrap them in warm, dry blankets. If you are outside, try to shield them from the wind and cold ground.

Next, encourage them to drink warm, non-alcoholic beverages. Hot water, tea, or broth are excellent choices, as they help to raise body temperature from the inside. Avoid caffeinated drinks, as they can lead to dehydration. If the person is alert enough to eat, provide them with warm, high-energy foods like soup or oatmeal, which can help restore energy levels.

Do not apply direct heat to the person, such as heating pads or hot water bottles, as this can cause burns on the cold skin. Instead, focus on gradual warming. Place warm compresses on their neck, armpits, and groin, which can help circulate warmth through the core of the body. Monitor their condition closely; if they become unconscious or unresponsive, seek medical attention immediately.

Recognizing Frostbite

When it comes to frostbite, recognizing the early signs is crucial. Initially, the affected skin may feel very cold and painful. As frostbite progresses, the skin will change color, often becoming red or pale, and may develop a waxy appearance. If you notice these changes, act quickly.

Examine the person's extremities, particularly the fingers, toes, and ears. If you notice blisters, or if the skin feels hard or numb, frostbite has likely occurred. In severe cases, the skin may turn black, indicating tissue death.

Responding to Frostbite

If someone has frostbite, it's essential to warm the affected areas gradually. Start by moving them to a warm environment. Avoid rubbing the affected skin, as this can cause more damage. Instead, gently soak the frostbitten area in warm (not hot) water for 30 to 40 minutes. Make sure the water is comfortable to the touch for non-affected skin.

After soaking, gently dry the skin with a soft towel and cover it with loose, dry cloths. Avoid breaking any blisters that may form; these protect the underlying skin and should be left intact if possible. If you notice any signs of infection, such as increased redness, swelling, or discharge, seek medical help.

If the frostbite is severe and the skin has turned black, do not attempt to rewarm the affected area; this can cause more damage. Seek immediate medical assistance.

Extra Tips for Prevention and Management

Preventing hypothermia and frostbite is just as important as knowing how to treat them. Dress in layers to keep your body warm and dry. Use waterproof and windproof outer layers to protect against the elements. Always wear hats, gloves, and warm socks, as a significant amount of body heat is lost through the head and extremities.

Stay hydrated and well-fed when spending time outdoors in the cold. Eating high-energy foods can help maintain your body temperature. Additionally, take regular breaks to warm up, especially if you start feeling cold.

Preventing Weather-Related Illnesses

Extreme weather conditions can significantly impact your health. Whether it's the intense heat of summer or the biting cold of winter, understanding how to prevent weather-related illnesses is crucial for everyone, especially those with underlying health conditions, children, and the elderly. By being proactive and informed, you can take steps to ensure that you and your loved ones stay safe and healthy during adverse weather conditions. This section will provide practical advice on how to prevent illnesses caused by extreme heat, cold, and other weather-related factors.

When dealing with extreme heat, it's essential to be aware of the risks associated with heat exhaustion and heatstroke. Heat exhaustion can occur when your body loses excessive amounts of water and salt through sweating. Symptoms may include heavy sweating, weakness, dizziness, nausea, and even fainting. To prevent heat-related illnesses, it's vital to stay hydrated. Drink plenty of water throughout the day, even if you don't feel thirsty. Limit your intake of alcohol and caffeine, as they can lead to dehydration.

It's also important to plan your outdoor activities during the cooler parts of the day. Try to avoid strenuous activities during peak heat hours, usually between 10 a.m. and 4 p.m. If you must be outside, wear loose-fitting, lightweight clothing in light colors. Dark colors can absorb heat, making you feel hotter. Additionally, don't forget to apply sunscreen to protect your skin from sunburn, which can add to heat stress.

If you notice someone showing signs of heat exhaustion, it's crucial to act quickly. Move the person to a cooler location, ideally air-conditioned, and have them lie down. Offer them water or a sports drink to help replenish lost fluids and electrolytes. If symptoms worsen or do not improve within 30 minutes, seek medical attention immediately.

When it comes to extreme cold, the risks of hypothermia and frostbite are serious. Hypothermia occurs when the body loses heat faster than it can produce it, leading to dangerously low body temperatures. Symptoms can include shivering, confusion, fatigue, and slurred speech. Frostbite, on the other hand, is damage to skin and underlying tissues caused by freezing. It's most commonly seen on the nose, fingers, and toes.

To prevent cold-related illnesses, dress in layers. This allows you to adjust your clothing to maintain a comfortable body temperature. Your outer layer should be windproof and waterproof to keep out moisture. Wear a hat and gloves, as a significant amount of body heat is lost through the head and extremities. Be mindful of the wind chill factor, which can make it feel much colder than the actual temperature.

Limit your time outdoors during extreme cold, and take frequent breaks indoors to warm up. Keep an eye out for signs of hypothermia or frostbite in yourself and others. If someone shows signs of hypothermia, move them to a warmer place, remove any wet clothing, and cover them with warm blankets. Offer warm drinks if they are conscious and alert, but avoid alcohol, as it can lower body temperature.

In addition to heat and cold, other weather-related factors can affect health. For instance, during periods of high humidity, heat-related illnesses can be exacerbated. High humidity levels make it harder for sweat to evaporate, reducing your body's ability to cool itself. If you're in a high-humidity area, consider spending time in air-conditioned spaces and taking frequent breaks from outdoor activities.

Air quality is another important consideration, especially during the summer when pollution levels can rise. Stay informed about air quality reports, especially if you or someone you care for has respiratory issues. On days when air quality is poor, limit outdoor activities, especially strenuous ones. If you must go outside, consider wearing a mask to filter out pollutants.

Additionally, severe weather events, like storms and hurricanes, can pose their own health risks. If a storm is approaching, make sure to stock up on necessary supplies, including food, water, and first aid supplies. Having an emergency kit ready can significantly reduce the stress and health risks associated with severe weather.

When planning for weather-related illnesses, consider these tips. Stay informed about the weather conditions in your area through local news and weather apps. Educate yourself and your family about the symptoms of heat-related and cold-related illnesses, so you can recognize them early. Create a plan for outdoor activities that considers the temperature and humidity levels.

Having a buddy system can also be effective—check in on friends, family, or neighbors who may be at risk during extreme weather. Make sure everyone in your household knows how to respond in case of an emergency, including how to perform first aid if someone becomes ill due to weather conditions.

By being proactive and aware of the risks associated with extreme weather, you can take the necessary steps to keep yourself and your loved ones safe. Remember that prevention is key to avoiding weather-related illnesses.

Extra Tips:

-Keep a thermometer handy to monitor body temperature in extreme conditions.

-If you're traveling, familiarize yourself with the climate of your destination.

-Regularly check on elderly neighbors or those with chronic conditions during extreme weather.

-Have a first aid kit accessible, complete with necessary supplies for treating heat-related and cold-related illnesses.

Chapter 12: Bites and Stings

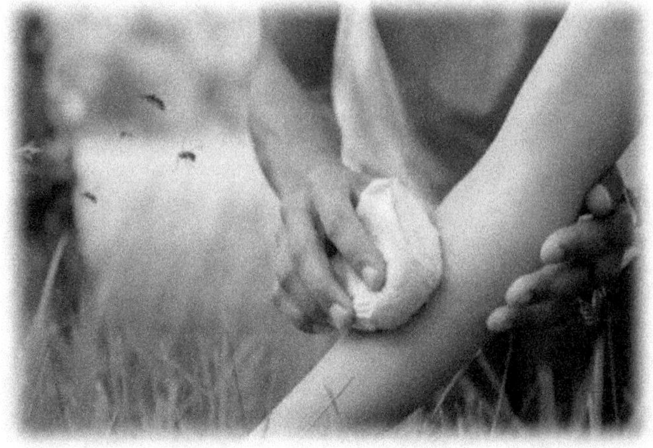

While on vacation, 10-year-old Emma was stung by a jellyfish. Her parents, unaware of proper first aid, attempted to rinse the sting with freshwater and applied heat. Unbeknownst to them, this exacerbated the venom's spread. Emma's condition rapidly deteriorated, leading to severe swelling, respiratory distress, and a prolonged hospital stay. The potentially life-threatening complications could have been avoided if her parents had known to rinse the sting with saltwater, remove tentacles, and seek immediate medical attention.

First Aid for Insect Bites and Stings

Insect bites and stings are common occurrences that can happen to anyone, anywhere. Understanding how to respond quickly and effectively can help reduce pain, prevent complications, and ensure a swift recovery. Whether it's a mosquito bite or a bee sting, knowing the right steps to take is essential for effective first aid.

When you or someone around you gets bitten or stung, the first thing to do is to remain calm. Most insect bites and stings are not serious and can be treated at home. However, it's important to recognize the symptoms and take appropriate action, especially if there are signs of an allergic reaction.

Identifying the Bite or Sting

Different insects leave different reactions, so identifying the type of bite or sting can guide your treatment. Mosquito bites typically cause itchy, raised welts on the skin. Flea bites may appear as small red bumps, often in clusters, particularly around the ankles and lower legs. Tick bites can be more serious due to the potential for Lyme disease and may require careful removal. On the other hand, bee and wasp stings can cause immediate pain, swelling, and redness at the site of the sting.

Initial Response

If someone is bitten or stung, start by assessing the situation. Check for any immediate allergic reactions, such as difficulty breathing, swelling of the face or throat, or rapid heartbeat. If any of these symptoms occur, seek emergency medical help immediately.

For minor bites and stings without severe reactions, follow these steps:

1. **Clean the Area**: Use soap and water to gently clean the bite or sting area. This step helps to reduce the risk of infection.

2. **Apply a Cold Compress**: To minimize swelling and numb the pain, apply a cold

compress or ice wrapped in a cloth to the affected area. Leave it on for about 10 to 15 minutes. Avoid applying ice directly to the skin, as it can cause frostbite.

3. Take Pain Relief: Over-the-counter pain relief medications, such as ibuprofen or acetaminophen, can help alleviate pain and discomfort. Follow the dosage instructions on the label for safe use.

4. Use Antihistamines: If itching or swelling is significant, consider using an antihistamine, such as diphenhydramine (Benadryl). This can help reduce allergic reactions and relieve itching. Always read the label for proper dosing, especially for children.

5. Monitor the Bite or Sting: Keep an eye on the affected area over the next few hours. If the pain increases, if there are signs of infection (like increasing redness, warmth, or pus), or if any severe allergic symptoms develop, seek medical attention.

Treating Specific Bites and Stings

In addition to the general first aid steps, here are some specific treatments for common insect bites and stings:

Bee Stings: If you are stung by a bee, the stinger may still be in your skin. Carefully remove the stinger as soon as possible using a flat object like a credit card. Avoid pinching it, as this can release more venom. Clean the area and follow the steps outlined above.

Fire Ant Stings: Fire ant stings can be particularly painful and often result in a blistering reaction. Clean the area and apply a topical antibiotic ointment to prevent infection. Monitor for any signs of allergic reaction.

Spider Bites: Most spider bites are harmless, but bites from black widows or brown recluses can be serious. Clean the bite and seek medical attention immediately if you suspect a dangerous spider bite.

Tick Bites: For tick bites, carefully remove the tick with fine-tipped tweezers, grasping it as close to the skin's surface as possible. Pull upward with steady, even pressure. After removal, clean the area with rubbing alcohol or soap and water. Watch for symptoms of Lyme disease, like a rash or fever, and consult a healthcare professional if they occur.

When to Seek Medical Attention

While most insect bites and stings can be treated at home, certain situations require immediate medical care. If you observe any of the following, act quickly:

-Signs of anaphylaxis, which can include difficulty breathing, swelling of the face or throat, a rapid pulse, or dizziness.

-Symptoms of infection at the bite or sting site, such as increasing redness, warmth, swelling, or pus.

-If a tick remains embedded in the skin after removal or if a rash develops afterward.

-Persistent pain, swelling, or fever that lasts longer than a couple of days.

Extra Tips

To prevent insect bites and stings, wear protective clothing, use insect repellent when outdoors, and avoid areas known for high insect activity. If you know you are allergic to insect stings, carry an epinephrine auto-injector (EpiPen) and know how to use it. Always inform family and friends about your allergies to ensure they can help in an emergency.

Understanding how to respond to insect bites and stings can make a significant difference in your and others' safety and comfort. By following these first aid steps and knowing when to seek help, you can handle these common situations with confidence.

Treating Animal Bites and Snake Bites

Animal bites and snake bites can be alarming situations that require prompt attention. Understanding how to manage these incidents is essential for minimizing harm and ensuring proper recovery. When faced with an animal bite, whether from a pet or a wild animal, it's crucial to assess the injury's severity and take appropriate steps. Similarly, snake bites can pose significant risks, depending on the type of snake involved. This guide will help you navigate these situations with confidence and clarity, ensuring you know what to do when these emergencies arise.

When you encounter an animal bite, the first step is to evaluate the wound. Look for signs of bleeding, swelling, or infection. If the bite has broken the skin, it's essential to control any bleeding. Apply gentle pressure with a clean cloth or bandage. If the bleeding is severe and does not stop after a few minutes, seek medical attention immediately. For minor bites, you can usually manage the injury at home.

After addressing any bleeding, it's important to clean the wound thoroughly. Rinse the bite area under clean running water for at least 5 to 10 minutes. This helps remove dirt, bacteria, and saliva that could lead to infection. Once the area is clean, gently pat it dry with a clean towel. Avoid using alcohol or hydrogen peroxide, as these can irritate the skin and delay healing.

Next, you'll want to apply an over-the-counter antibiotic ointment to help prevent infection. After applying the ointment, cover the bite with a sterile bandage. Keep the wound clean and dry, and change the dressing daily or if it becomes wet or dirty. It's essential to monitor the wound for signs of infection, which can include increased redness, swelling, warmth, or pus. If you notice any of these symptoms, seek medical help promptly.

In some cases, animal bites may require a tetanus shot, especially if the bitten person has not had one in the last five years. Tetanus is a serious infection caused by bacteria that can enter the body through wounds. If the bite is deep or from an unknown animal, it's essential to consult a healthcare professional for advice on tetanus immunization and the need for further treatment.

Additionally, it's crucial to identify the animal that caused the bite. If the animal is a pet, you should contact the owner to determine if the pet is up to date on vaccinations, particularly rabies. Rabies is a deadly virus transmitted through saliva, and bites from rabid animals can pose a serious health threat. If the animal is wild or cannot be identified, medical professionals may recommend a rabies vaccination as a precaution.

When it comes to snake bites, the first thing you need to do is remain calm. Panic can raise your heart rate and spread venom more quickly through the bloodstream. Move away from the snake to avoid further bites and call for emergency help. If you are with the victim, keep them as still as possible to slow the spread of venom.

While waiting for medical assistance, you can take some steps to help manage the situation. If possible, keep the affected limb immobilized and at or below heart level to reduce the spread of venom. Do not apply ice or a tourniquet, as these can worsen tissue damage and complications. Avoid cutting the bite site or attempting to suck out the venom. These methods are not effective and can lead to additional injuries or infections.

If you know the type of snake that bit the person, provide that information to the medical team when they arrive. If it's safe to do so, take a picture of the snake, or remember its colors and patterns. This information can help healthcare providers determine the appropriate treatment.

Upon receiving medical attention, healthcare professionals may administer antivenom if the snake is venomous. They will also monitor the patient for signs of an allergic reaction or complications from the bite. Follow any aftercare instructions provided by the medical team, including any prescribed medications.

Here are a few extra tips to keep in mind: Always wash your hands before and after treating any wounds to prevent infection. Educate yourself and your family about local wildlife, including which snakes are venomous in your area, to reduce the risk of bites. Lastly, consider taking a first aid course to better prepare yourself for emergencies, so you can handle such situations with confidence.

Managing Allergic Reactions to Bites and Stings

Allergic reactions to bites and stings can range from mild irritation to severe, life-threatening conditions. Understanding how to recognize and manage these reactions is crucial for the safety of both children and adults. This section will guide you through the signs of allergic reactions, the steps to take for management, and the appropriate first aid responses to ensure safety and comfort.

Allergic reactions occur when the immune system mistakenly identifies a harmless substance, like venom from a bee sting or proteins in an insect bite, as a threat. This results in the release of histamines and other chemicals that can cause various symptoms. Not everyone will have the same response to a bite or sting, which makes it important to be vigilant and informed.

When managing an allergic reaction, first, be on the lookout for common symptoms. These can include redness, swelling, itching, or hives around the bite or sting site. In more severe cases, individuals may experience difficulty breathing, swelling of the face or throat, rapid heartbeat, dizziness, or even loss of consciousness. Recognizing these signs early can make a significant difference in how you respond.

If you suspect someone is having an allergic reaction, the first step is to ensure their safety. If they have a known allergy and carry an epinephrine auto-injector, assist them in using it immediately. Inject the epinephrine into the outer thigh, holding it in place for a few seconds to ensure the medication is delivered. This can help reverse severe symptoms and provide critical time until emergency help arrives.

In addition to administering epinephrine, it's important to assess the bite or sting site. Remove any stingers that may be lodged in the skin by gently scraping the area with a flat-edged object like a credit card. Avoid pinching the stinger, as this can release more venom. After the stinger is removed, wash the area with soap and water to prevent infection. Pat the area dry and apply a cold compress to reduce swelling and provide relief from pain and itching.

For mild reactions, you may treat the symptoms at home. Over-the-counter antihistamines like diphenhydramine (Benadryl) can help reduce itching and swelling. Always follow the dosing instructions on the label, especially when administering to children. Additionally, applying hydrocortisone cream can soothe irritation. It's essential to keep the area clean and monitor for any changes. If symptoms worsen or do not improve, seek medical advice.

If the person is experiencing difficulty breathing or shows signs of anaphylaxis—such as swelling in the throat, a rapid pulse, or confusion—call emergency services immediately. While waiting for help, keep the individual calm and in a comfortable position. Lying down with their feet elevated can help with blood circulation if they feel faint. Do not give them anything to eat or drink, as this could cause choking if they are having difficulty breathing.

Education plays a vital role in managing allergic reactions. Ensure that individuals who are prone to allergic responses have a clear action plan and are aware of their triggers. Teach them to recognize the symptoms and understand the importance of prompt action. Encourage them to inform friends, family, and caregivers about their allergies so that everyone knows how to help in case of an emergency.

In addition to knowing how to respond to bites and stings, taking preventive measures can significantly reduce the risk of allergic reactions. Wearing long sleeves and pants in areas where insects are prevalent can minimize exposure. Using insect repellent containing DEET or other approved ingredients can deter insect bites. It's also wise to avoid brightly colored clothing or floral patterns, which can attract bees and other insects.

Finally, keep a well-stocked first aid kit on hand, including items specifically for treating allergic reactions. This should contain antihistamines, an epinephrine auto-injector if prescribed, antiseptic wipes, and hydrocortisone cream. Familiarize yourself with the kit so you can quickly access what you need in an emergency.

By knowing how to manage allergic reactions to bites and stings, you can ensure a safer environment for yourself and those around you. Being prepared and informed is key to effectively responding to these situations, helping to prevent complications and ensuring everyone can enjoy outdoor activities with confidence.

Extra Tips:

Always carry an allergy card detailing any known allergies, including what to do in case of an emergency. Consider taking a first aid and

CPR class to further enhance your skills and confidence in handling allergic reactions and other medical emergencies.

Chapter 13: First Aid for Heart-Related Emergencies

When 55-year-old David suddenly clutched his chest in pain, his wife, Susan, panicked and drove him to the hospital instead of calling 911. Valuable time was lost, and by the time they arrived, David's heart attack had progressed, causing irreversible damage. Despite medical intervention, David suffered severe heart damage, significantly impacting his quality of life. Susan later learned that prompt recognition of heart attack symptoms and timely administration of CPR and emergency medical services could have greatly improved David's outcome.

Recognizing the Signs of a Heart Attack

Understanding how to recognize the signs of a heart attack is crucial for saving lives. A heart attack, medically known as a myocardial infarction, occurs when blood flow to a part of the heart is blocked, usually by a blood clot. Quick recognition and response can significantly improve the chances of survival and recovery. This section will guide you through the common signs of a heart attack, helping you identify when someone might be in serious danger.

When it comes to heart attacks, people often think of chest pain as the primary symptom. While chest pain is indeed a significant sign, it's essential to remember that heart attacks can present in various ways, and not everyone experiences the same symptoms. Understanding these can help you take action promptly.

One of the most common symptoms is discomfort or pain in the center or left side of the chest. This sensation might feel like a pressure, squeezing, fullness, or an aching feeling. Some individuals describe it as a heavy weight resting on their chest. It can come and go, lasting for a few minutes, or it may persist. If you notice someone experiencing this kind of discomfort, it's critical to pay attention, especially if it's accompanied by other signs.

Apart from chest pain, many people experience discomfort in other areas of the upper body. This discomfort can radiate to the arms, particularly the left arm, but it can also spread to the back, neck, jaw, or stomach. For example, someone might feel a dull ache in their jaw or experience a tightness in their back. This can make it tricky to identify a heart attack since these symptoms can also be related to other conditions. Encourage individuals experiencing such discomfort to seek medical attention immediately.

Shortness of breath is another vital sign to look for. This can occur with or without chest discomfort. A person may feel like they can't catch their breath or are struggling to breathe, which can lead to feelings of anxiety. If someone exhibits this symptom, it is essential to assess their condition quickly. Often, shortness of breath may present itself during physical activity or even while resting.

Other signs that might indicate a heart attack include cold sweat, nausea, or lightheadedness. Some people report feeling unusually sweaty, as if they have just finished an intense workout, while others may experience stomach discomfort or vomiting. Lightheadedness can lead to fainting, so it's crucial to ensure the person stays safe and seated if they exhibit these symptoms.

Women, in particular, may experience different signs than men. While chest pain is still common, women are more likely to report symptoms such as fatigue, sleep disturbances, and anxiety. They might also feel back or jaw pain more frequently than men do. It's vital not to dismiss these signs, especially in women, as they can often go unnoticed and be mistaken for stress or other non-life-threatening issues.

Recognizing these signs can empower you to act quickly. If you suspect that someone is having a heart attack, do not wait to see if the symptoms pass. Call emergency services immediately. Provide the operator with as much information as possible about the person's symptoms and condition. If the person is conscious and alert, encourage them to chew and swallow an aspirin if they're not allergic to it. Aspirin can help thin the blood and improve blood flow to the heart, but it should only be given if it's safe for the individual.

While waiting for emergency medical help to arrive, it's essential to keep the person calm. If they are conscious, have them sit or lie down in a comfortable position. Stress and anxiety can exacerbate symptoms, so reassuring them can be incredibly beneficial. Monitor their condition closely. If they lose consciousness or stop breathing, be prepared to perform CPR until professional help arrives.

Understanding and recognizing the signs of a heart attack can make a difference. Your ability to act quickly could save someone's life. It's vital to remember that even if you are unsure, it's better to err on the side of caution. Taking quick action can provide the affected person with the best chance of recovery.

Extra Tips

If you or someone you know is at higher risk for heart disease, such as those with a family history of heart problems, high blood pressure, or diabetes, it's wise to stay informed about heart health. Regular check-ups and discussions with a healthcare provider about any concerning symptoms are vital. Knowing your own body and recognizing changes can also help in identifying potential heart issues early on. Lastly, encouraging healthy lifestyle choices, like a balanced diet, regular exercise, and avoiding smoking, can significantly reduce the risk of heart attacks in the long run.

Administering First Aid for a Stroke

Recognizing and responding to a stroke quickly can make a significant difference in a person's recovery. Understanding how to administer first aid for a stroke is crucial, as every minute counts. This section will guide you through the signs of a stroke, the steps to take immediately, and how to support the individual until medical professionals arrive.

A stroke occurs when there is an interruption of blood flow to the brain, which can lead to brain damage and other complications. The two main types of strokes are ischemic, caused by a blockage in a blood vessel, and hemorrhagic, resulting from a burst blood vessel. Knowing the signs and how to respond can save lives and minimize long-term effects.

Recognizing the Signs of a Stroke

The first step in administering first aid is recognizing the signs of a stroke. The acronym

FAST can help you remember the key symptoms to watch for:

-**Face Drooping**: Ask the person to smile. Does one side of their face droop or feel numb?

-**Arm Weakness**: Ask them to raise both arms. Does one arm drift downward or feel weak?

-**Speech Difficulty**: Ask the person to repeat a simple phrase. Is their speech slurred or hard to understand?

-**Time to Call Emergency Services**: If you notice any of these signs, it's essential to seek immediate medical help. Do not wait to see if symptoms go away.

What to Do in an Emergency

Once you recognize that someone is having a stroke, follow these steps:

1. **Call for Help**: Dial emergency services immediately. Provide clear information about the situation, including the person's symptoms

and the time they first appeared. This information is crucial for medical professionals.

2. Keep the Person Calm: Reassure the individual that help is on the way. Encourage them to stay as calm as possible and avoid any unnecessary movement. Try to keep them in a comfortable position, typically lying down with their head slightly elevated.

3. Monitor Their Condition: While waiting for emergency services, keep a close eye on the person's condition. Check their breathing and responsiveness. If they become unconscious and do not have a pulse, be prepared to start CPR if you're trained to do so.

4. Positioning: If the person is conscious, place them in a safe position, preferably on their side to help with breathing and prevent choking if they vomit. If they're unconscious, ensure they are lying on their side in the recovery position.

5. Do Not Give Food or Drink: Avoid giving the person any food, drink, or medication.

Swallowing may be compromised during a stroke, increasing the risk of choking.

Providing Support after the Initial Response

Once emergency services arrive, provide them with any information they may need about the person's condition and the symptoms you observed. Be prepared to answer questions about their medical history, any medications they take, and when the symptoms began.

Understanding Risk Factors and Prevention

It's also important to be aware of the risk factors that can lead to a stroke. High blood pressure, diabetes, high cholesterol, smoking, and a sedentary lifestyle can all increase the likelihood of a stroke. Encourage the individual and their family to consult with healthcare professionals about lifestyle changes and preventive measures.

Long-Term Care and Support

After the immediate first aid response, ongoing support and care will be necessary for the individual recovering from a stroke.

Rehabilitation can include physical therapy, occupational therapy, and speech therapy. Support from family and friends can play a vital role in recovery. Being patient and understanding the challenges they may face will greatly assist in their rehabilitation process.

Extra Tips for Stroke Awareness

1. Educate yourself and others: Learning the signs of a stroke and sharing this knowledge can help create a community that responds effectively in emergencies.

2. Regular Health Check-ups: Encourage regular health screenings to monitor and manage risk factors like blood pressure and cholesterol levels.

3. Maintain a Healthy Lifestyle: Promoting a balanced diet, regular exercise, and avoiding smoking can significantly reduce the risk of stroke.

4. Emergency Plan: Have an emergency plan in place that includes knowing who to contact and where to go in case of a medical emergency.

Administering first aid for a stroke requires prompt action and understanding. By recognizing the signs and knowing how to respond, you can be a vital support in a critical situation, ensuring that the affected person receives the help they need as quickly as possible.

Managing Sudden Cardiac Arrest

Sudden cardiac arrest (SCA) is a critical emergency that occurs when the heart unexpectedly stops beating. This can happen to anyone, regardless of age or health status, and it often leads to death if immediate action is not taken. Understanding how to respond effectively is vital, as your quick response can save a life. In this section, you will learn how to recognize sudden cardiac arrest, perform CPR, and use an Automated External Defibrillator (AED), ensuring that you are prepared to act in a crisis.

Recognizing sudden cardiac arrest is the first crucial step in managing the situation. The person experiencing SCA will suddenly collapse, become unresponsive, and will not be breathing or will be gasping. It's important to check for responsiveness by shaking the person gently and shouting, "Are you okay?" If there is no response and the person is not breathing normally, you need to act immediately.

Once you confirm that someone is in cardiac arrest, call for emergency medical assistance right away. If you are alone, call for help before starting CPR. If others are present, instruct someone to call emergency services while you begin resuscitation efforts. Time is critical, as every minute without oxygen increases the risk of permanent damage or death.

Begin CPR as soon as possible. This involves two main components: chest compressions and rescue breaths. If you are trained in CPR, start with chest compressions. Position the heel of one hand on the center of the person's chest and place the other hand on top. Keep your arms straight and use your body weight to push down hard and fast, compressing the chest to a depth of about two inches at a rate of 100 to 120 compressions per minute. Allow the chest to rise completely between compressions. This rhythm can be matched to the beat of a song like "Stayin'

Alive" by the Bee Gees, which can help you maintain the correct pace.

After 30 compressions, if you are trained and feel comfortable doing so, give two rescue breaths. To do this, tilt the person's head back slightly to open the airway, pinch their nose shut, and give a breath that lasts about one second. Watch for the chest to rise. Then, give a second breath in the same manner. Continue the cycle of 30 chest compressions followed by two rescue breaths until emergency help arrives or the person starts to show signs of life, such as breathing normally or moving.

If an AED is available, use it as soon as possible. These devices are designed to be user-friendly and provide voice prompts to guide you through the process. Turn on the AED and follow the visual and audio instructions provided. Typically, you will need to expose the person's chest and attach the pads as indicated on the device. One pad goes on the upper right side of the chest, and the other goes on the lower left side.

Once the pads are placed, the AED will analyze the heart's rhythm. If a shock is advised, ensure that no one is touching the person, and press the button to deliver the shock. After the shock is given, or if no shock is advised, resume CPR immediately. Continue this cycle of CPR and using the AED until emergency responders arrive.

To enhance your readiness for emergencies involving sudden cardiac arrest, consider these extra tips:

1. **Get trained**: Taking a CPR and AED certification course will prepare you to respond confidently in emergencies. Many organizations, such as the Red Cross and American Heart Association, offer training sessions.

2. **Have an AED accessible**: If you are in a public space, familiarize yourself with the

location of the nearest AED. In your home or workplace, consider purchasing an AED for easy access during emergencies.

3. Stay calm: In high-pressure situations, it's natural to feel anxious. Take a deep breath and focus on following the steps you've learned. Your ability to remain calm can significantly impact your effectiveness.

4. Encourage others to get trained: Spread the word about the importance of first aid training. The more people who are prepared to respond, the better the chances of survival for someone experiencing sudden cardiac arrest.

By equipping yourself with knowledge and skills, you can make a difference when every moment counts. Remember that your actions may help save a life in a critical situation.

Chapter 14: Emergency Childbirth

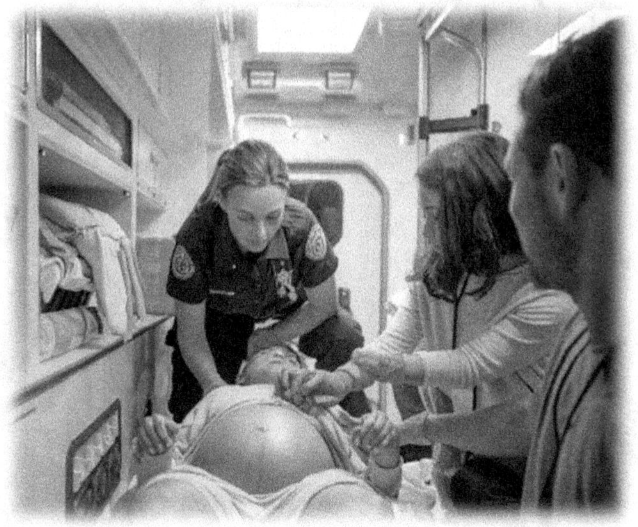

When 25-year-old Rihanna went into sudden labor, her friend, Rachel, unaware of emergency childbirth procedures, attempted to drive her to the hospital. Delayed arrival and lack of proper prenatal care resulted in complications, causing Rihanna to give birth in the car. The umbilical cord was wrapped around the baby's neck, and without proper intervention, the newborn suffered oxygen deprivation, leading to lifelong developmental delays. Had Rachel known basic emergency childbirth techniques, such as calling 911 and providing adequate care until medical help arrived, the outcome might have been vastly different.

Recognizing Signs of Imminent Childbirth

When you're in a situation where someone is about to give birth, it's crucial to recognize the signs of imminent childbirth. This knowledge can help you provide the right assistance and ensure the safety of both the mother and the baby. In this section, we'll explore the key indicators that labor is starting and how you can prepare for what comes next.

The signs that indicate imminent childbirth can vary from person to person, but there are several common physical and emotional cues you can watch for. Knowing these signs can help you respond effectively and calmly.

One of the primary signs that labor is starting is the onset of regular contractions. These contractions are typically felt as a tightening or cramping in the abdomen. Early on, they may be spaced far apart, but as labor progresses, they will become more frequent and intense. You can help the mother track these contractions by timing their duration and frequency. Generally, if contractions occur every five minutes and last for at least a minute, this can indicate that labor is progressing rapidly.

Another sign to watch for is the rupture of the amniotic sac, often referred to as "water breaking." This event can happen before labor begins or during the early stages of labor. When the water breaks, a clear or pale yellow fluid may leak from the vagina. If this occurs, it's essential to note the time, as this can impact how the delivery is managed. If the fluid is green or brown, it may indicate the presence of meconium, which can pose risks to the baby, so alert medical personnel immediately.

You might also notice physical changes in the mother that indicate she is in labor. These can include a change in her breathing pattern, increased anxiety, or even nesting behavior, where she suddenly feels a strong urge to prepare her environment for the baby. Additionally, as the baby moves down the birth canal, you may observe that the mother's belly appears to "drop." This is known as lightening and can happen a few weeks or days before labor starts.

Emotional signs can be just as telling. The mother may exhibit a mix of excitement, anxiety, and focus as she prepares for childbirth. It's essential to offer your support during this time. Keeping the atmosphere calm and reassuring can help her feel more at ease. Encourage her to breathe deeply and stay hydrated, as this can help ease some of the discomfort associated with labor.

Another key indicator of imminent childbirth is the presence of the "bloody show," which refers to a mixture of blood and mucus that can be discharged from the vagina as the cervix begins to dilate. This usually occurs as the body prepares for labor, and it's a sign that things are progressing. If you see this, it's a good idea to monitor the timing of contractions, as it can indicate that labor is nearing.

As labor progresses, you might observe the mother experiencing a change in her ability to communicate. She may become less talkative, focusing instead on managing her contractions. This shift can indicate that the labor is advancing and that delivery may be imminent. It's important to respect her space while also being ready to assist her as needed.

In any case, recognizing these signs is just the beginning. Once you identify that the mother is likely going into labor, you should ensure that you have a plan in place. Make sure you know the quickest route to the nearest medical facility or have the necessary contact information for emergency services. If you have time, gather supplies that may be needed, such as clean towels, blankets, and a first aid kit.

If it becomes evident that the baby is about to be born, it's crucial to be prepared for delivery. Find a clean and safe area for the mother to lie down. Ensure that she is as comfortable as possible, and help her maintain a position that feels natural to her, whether it's lying on her side, sitting, or even squatting.

As you wait for help to arrive, reassure her that she is doing great. Encourage her to breathe through the contractions, and remind her that she is close to meeting her baby. This emotional support can be invaluable during such a pivotal moment.

Remember to stay calm and collected throughout the process.

Extra Tips:

-Familiarize yourself with local emergency numbers and the nearest hospital.

-Keep a small bag prepared with essential items for emergencies.

-Encourage the mother to practice relaxation techniques, which can help her cope better during labor.

-If you're in a public place, alert nearby staff to ensure they can assist when necessary.

-Stay flexible and adaptable, as childbirth can be unpredictable.

Assisting in a Delivery in an Emergency Situation

When faced with the unexpected event of assisting in a delivery, it's essential to remain calm and focused. While giving birth is usually a process managed by healthcare professionals, emergencies can arise when help is not immediately available. Understanding the basic steps involved in assisting a delivery can help ensure the safety of both the mother and the baby during this critical time.

First, assess the situation. If a woman is in labor and unable to reach a hospital, or if the baby is coming too quickly, you need to act promptly. Ensure that the environment is safe and comfortable. If possible, have the woman lie down in a position that feels most comfortable for her, typically on her back with knees bent or on her side. It's important to keep her as relaxed as possible to facilitate the delivery.

Before the actual delivery begins, gather supplies. You will need clean towels or cloths, a sterile surface if possible, and a clean pair of scissors (if cutting the umbilical cord is necessary). If available, have gloves on hand to maintain hygiene. Ensure that your hands are clean, and wash them thoroughly with soap and water or use hand sanitizer if soap isn't available.

Next, you should monitor the contractions. Contractions will indicate how close the baby is to being delivered. Timing the contractions can help you gauge how quickly you need to proceed. If the contractions are close together, it's a sign that the baby may be arriving soon. Encourage the mother to breathe deeply and relax during each contraction. You can help by counting with her, guiding her through breathing techniques that promote calmness.

As the baby begins to descend, you may notice the mother experiencing increased pressure. This is the time when she may feel the urge to push. Encourage her to follow her instincts. If she feels the need to push, she should do so during a contraction. Remind her to take deep breaths in between contractions to keep her energy up.

When the baby's head starts to crown, this is a critical moment. You may see the top of the head beginning to emerge. It's essential to support the head gently as it comes out, guiding it with your hands while allowing the mother to push. Once the head is delivered, you will see the umbilical cord. Do not attempt to pull the baby out; let the mother continue pushing naturally.

After the head is out, the shoulders will follow. Place your hands on the baby's shoulders, ready to gently guide the rest of the body as it is delivered. Ensure that you are supporting the baby and not pulling on it, as this can cause injury. As soon as the baby is fully delivered, you need to dry and wrap the baby in clean towels to help regulate body temperature and stimulate breathing.

Next, check to see if the umbilical cord is wrapped around the baby's neck. If it is, gently slip it over the baby's head if possible. If you cannot do this, don't panic. Just keep the baby supported, and allow emergency personnel to handle this when they arrive.

Once the baby is out and stable, turn your attention to the mother. Help her into a comfortable position, usually with her legs bent and resting. Encourage her to take slow, deep breaths and reassure her that she is doing well. After the delivery, the placenta will need to be delivered, which usually happens naturally within a few minutes.

If the mother experiences excessive bleeding, apply gentle pressure to her abdomen, and encourage her to breastfeed if possible, as this can help the uterus contract. Monitor the mother's condition closely and be prepared to provide additional support as needed. If she feels faint or lightheaded, have her lie down and elevate her legs to improve blood flow.

After everything is stabilized, continue to provide comfort to both the mother and the baby until help arrives. Keep talking to them, reassuring them, and providing any necessary assistance.

Extra Tips:

-Always prioritize safety; if you feel overwhelmed or unsure, try to contact emergency services as soon as possible.

-Encourage the mother to trust her instincts throughout the process.

-Stay calm and composed, as your demeanor can significantly impact the mother's stress levels.

-If possible, have someone else call for help while you assist with the delivery.

-Remember, every birth is different, so be flexible and adapt to the situation as it unfolds.

First Aid for Newborns: Clearing Airways and Managing Complications

When a newborn arrives, the first moments can be both joyful and nerve-wracking, especially if complications arise. Understanding how to clear airways and manage issues effectively is crucial for ensuring your baby's safety and well-being. This guide provides essential information on handling these situations calmly and effectively, empowering you to respond when it matters most.

Newborns, especially those born prematurely or with health issues, may have difficulty breathing due to various reasons. It's essential to recognize signs of distress early. Signs include rapid breathing, grunting, flaring nostrils, or a bluish tint around the lips and face. If you notice these symptoms, it's critical to act quickly. Here's how to help clear the airways and manage potential complications.

Start by ensuring the newborn is lying on their back on a firm surface, such as a changing table or a bed. Always keep one hand on your baby to prevent falls. If the baby is crying, this is a good sign as it indicates they are breathing; however, if they seem to have difficulty making sounds or are silent, you may need to take immediate action.

Next, gently stimulate your baby. Sometimes, simply rubbing their back or tapping their feet can encourage them to breathe more easily. If the baby is still having trouble, it may be necessary to clear the airway.

To do this, you can use a bulb syringe. This tool is designed to gently suction mucus or other obstructions from your baby's nose and mouth. Start by squeezing the bulb to expel air, then gently insert the tip into one nostril while keeping the other nostril closed. Slowly release the bulb to create suction, which will draw out mucus. Remove the syringe and clean it before repeating on the other nostril. This method can help clear any blockage and allow the baby to breathe more comfortably.

Another method to consider is using saline drops. These can be helpful if your newborn has a lot of congestion. You can place one or two drops of saline into each nostril. Wait a few moments, then use the bulb syringe to suction again. This can help to loosen mucus and make it easier to remove.

If your newborn is still struggling to breathe after clearing the airways, you may need to perform a series of back blows and chest thrusts, but be cautious. For newborns, the technique differs slightly from that used for older children and adults. Place your baby face down on your forearm, supporting their head and neck. Use the heel of your other hand to deliver up to five gentle back blows between the shoulder blades. Be sure to keep your hand supporting the baby's head, and avoid excessive force. If this doesn't resolve the situation, turn your baby over and perform chest thrusts by placing two fingers in the center of the chest, just below the nipple line. Push down firmly and quickly, repeating this up to five times.

If your newborn shows no improvement after these steps, or if they become unresponsive, you need to call for emergency help immediately. While waiting for help to arrive, continue to monitor their breathing. If your baby is unresponsive, begin CPR, ensuring that you're familiar with the correct technique for infants. It's crucial to use gentle pressure and the appropriate rhythm to help your baby.

Aside from airway management, being aware of other potential complications is equally important. Newborns are susceptible to various conditions, including respiratory distress syndrome, which may occur due to underdeveloped lungs. Keep an eye out for persistent rapid breathing, retractions (where the skin pulls in around the ribs during inhalation), and nasal flaring. These symptoms require immediate medical attention.

In cases where a newborn is born with a congenital condition, such as congenital heart defects or tracheoesophageal fistula, understanding the specific first aid procedures is essential. Always consult your healthcare provider for personalized information on how to manage these situations based on your newborn's needs.

After any first aid intervention, make sure to follow up with a healthcare professional, even if the baby seems to recover. This is important for ensuring that there are no underlying issues that need addressing.

Extra Tips:

-Always keep emergency contact numbers handy, including your pediatrician and local emergency services.

-Consider taking a certified first aid and CPR course focused on infants and children to build your confidence.

-Familiarize yourself with your baby's breathing patterns so you can recognize any changes more easily.

-When in doubt, don't hesitate to seek help. It's better to be cautious than to risk your baby's health.

Conclusion

As we come to the conclusion of this first aid manual, you've taken a significant step in understanding the crucial skills needed to respond confidently to various emergencies. This book has guided you through essential first aid topics, from assessing situations to administering CPR, handling bleeding, managing fractures, treating burns, and much more. Each chapter has been designed to equip you with knowledge and methods that may one day be life-saving for you, your loved ones, or even strangers in need. Whether you're new to first aid or building upon previous knowledge, you now have a solid foundation to act with assurance and poise in critical moments.

To get the most from this book's content, here are some suggestions: Regularly revisit the material and review key techniques to keep them fresh in your mind. First aid skills are perishable, so reinforcing your understanding will ensure you're ready to respond when the need arises. If possible, consider practicing these techniques through hands-on courses or simulations, as practical experience will further enhance your confidence. Pairing this manual's information with certified training can give you an even more comprehensive skill set.

Don't underestimate the value of first aid practice with family, friends, or colleagues. Teaching others what you've learned will strengthen your knowledge while making the people around you more prepared in emergencies. By working together, you and your loved ones can build a support system to respond effectively to unexpected situations.

I want to remind you that your willingness to learn these skills already sets you apart. Emergencies are daunting, and it takes courage to be ready to face them head-on. Take pride in the fact that you're now equipped to help those around you in times of need. You're a part of a community of individuals dedicated to being prepared and proactive, contributing to safer and more resilient communities everywhere.

If this book has helped you, I would be incredibly grateful if you could leave a review. Your feedback not only helps future readers find the right resources but also supports the ongoing effort to spread first aid knowledge widely. Reviews play a vital role in reaching more people who may benefit from these life-saving techniques.

Be sure to explore my other books as well, where I cover a range of practical guides and how-to topics in areas like home improvement, family health, and emergency preparedness. Each book is crafted with the same commitment to clear, accessible information that empowers you to take control and make a difference in your world.

Thank you for choosing this manual, and for committing yourself to the vital knowledge of first aid. Remember, the skills you've learned are not just instructions on a page but tools for making a meaningful impact in critical moments. As you close this book, know that you've added something invaluable to your life—knowledge that could save a life. Wishing you confidence, calm, and strength in all your first aid efforts.